No Gallbladder Diet Cookbook

Essential Guide with 120 Delicious and Healthy Recipes & 30 Day Meal Plan for a Missing or Dysfunctional Gallbladder.

Thomas Miller

Table of Contents

Introduction

No gallbladder! What does that even mean? Is it possible to survive without a gallbladder? These are some of the most common series of questions asked by patients who have long been suffering from gallstones and their doctor's solution for the intense pain is the removal of their gallbladder.

However, what most people do not know is that you can lead a pain-free and perfectly normal life when your gallbladder is taken out. What happens to the bile produced by the liver? Well, your liver will continue with its task of secreting bile that is meant to digest the food you take the only difference once your gallbladder is taken out is that instead of this produced bile being stored in the gallbladder as it does in a person with a gallbladder, it drips little by little continuously into the digestive system.

In this no gallbladder diet guide we are going to be looking at what happens from the moment your doctor recommends a gallbladder removal surgery, also referred to as cholecystectomy; what happens and what you should do after the surgery and how to live a healthy life without a gallbladder. In the second part of this guide, we will look at a 30 day meal plan with 120 delicious recipes that are natural, super healthy and easy to prepare.

As you read this book, note down all the things you would like to discuss with your doctor in your next appointment, if you are yet to receive the surgery or if you are fresh from receiving the surgery to make your transition smoother.

If you have any pre-existing conditions, consult with your doctor on what you need to add and what you need to eliminate from your diet. The reason for this is that after your cholecystectomy, you will now be free to eat all the foods that you couldn't eat before because of the presence of gallstones.

With the right information, you can now make better informed choices as you endeavor to lead a healthy life and that's what you are going to get with this guide.

All the best!

Let's Start from the Beginning

The gall bladder is a tiny organ that has the shape of a pouch and is located right under your liver. The gall bladder stores the bile that is produced by your liver and it's essential for your biliary system. The liver is responsible for the production of bile which is necessary for digestion to take place. Your gallbladder goes on to hold onto this bile until your body requires to use it. While the gall bladder plays an important role in your body, it is not crucial to your survival as there are other ways of supplying bile to your small intestines. In fact, there are times when the gallbladder has to be surgically removed from your body in cases of serious presence of gallstones, gallbladder disease and gallbladder attack; which is what we are going to paying focus to in this diet guide.

The gallbladder acts as storage for bile and only releases it as needed for digestion. The absorbent lining of the gallbladder concentrates the bile. Once the food comes to your small intestine, cholecystokinin (a hormone) is released and this signals the gallbladder to secrete bile in the small intestines through a bile duct. The bile can break up digestive fats and eliminate waste products from your liver to your duodenum. For reasons that remain unclear, an imbalance of substances that make up bile can crystallize in your bladder and form gallstones. These are small and hard deposits in your gallbladder that resemble tiny stones hence the term gallstones. Most people are not able to identify the symptoms of small gallstones and only know there is a problem when the gallstones become enlarged when they start experiencing severe abdominal pain, inflammation or nausea.

Surgery to remove the gallbladder is usually recommended if you have severely painful gallstones. While most people are not even aware that they have gallstones, occasionally, these stones can obstruct the flow of bile which can lead to irritation of the gall bladder, a condition known as cholecystitis or irritation of the pancreas, a condition known as pancreatitis

These two conditions can result in:

- Jaundice

- Lethargy

- Sudden and extreme tummy pain

In some cases, it is possible to get medication that dissolves gallstones but ultimately, gallbladder removal surgery is the most effective form of treatment because here is no chance of recurring gallstones.

Gallbladder removal surgery

There are two main types of gallbladder removal surgeries and these are:

- An open cholecystectomy

In this form of surgery, a single incision is made on the stomach to gain access to the gallbladder which is then taken out.

- Keyhole or laparoscopic cholecystectomy

A number of tiny incisions are made on your stomach to gain access to your gallbladder which is then removed.

The most common form of surgery and the most recommended is the keyhole cholecystectomy as it allows a patient to leave the hospital faster, it has a quick recovery rate and the patient is left with very tiny scars compared to the open cholecystectomy.

Both of these surgery techniques are performed under general anesthesia meaning the patient doesn't feel a thing during the surgery.

What are the risks of gallbladder removal surgery?

A gallbladder removal surgery is considered to be one of the safest surgeries but that doesn't mean that it is immune from the risk of complications. Some possible complications that can arise from a gallbladder removal surgery are:

- Bile leakage into the stomach

When your surgeon takes out your gallbladder, they use special clips to fasten the tube that normally connect the main bile duct to the gallbladder. However, the bile fluid can occasional leak into the abdomen after your gallbladder has been removed.

The most common symptoms of a bile leak include severe abdominal pain, a distended stomach, high fever and feeling of lethargy.

- Damage to one of the ducts that transport bile from your liver

These ducts can get easily damaged during the cholecystectomy. If this happens when the surgery is taking place, the affected duct can be easily repaired. However, if the damaged duct(s) is identified after the surgery, another surgery will need to be done to fix it.

- Injury to blood vessels, intestines or bowel

- Formation of blood clots

Before undertaking a cholecystectomy, have a conversation with your surgeon about all the benefits and risks of the procedure you are about to undertake. Your doctor will recommend a preoperative assessment that will take place in the hospital several weeks leading to your scheduled surgery.

During this appointment, your doctor will discuss with you:

- Any concerns that you could be having and answer all the questions that come up.

- The results of the blood tests that will be carried out alongside a general checkup that are done to ensure that you are fit for surgery. The results are what will determine whether a keyhole cholecystectomy or an open cholecystectomy is best suited for you.

- When you are supposed to stop drinking and eating before your surgery.

- Some of the things you can do to reduce your risk of developing complications after your surgery such as not taking alcohol or smoking.

The Recovery Process

Just as mentioned, recovery from a keyhole cholecystectomy is quite fast and most patients often leave the hospital the same day of the surgery or latest, the next morning, unless complications arise.

It is usually possible to return to all your normal duties within a fortnight. However, in the case of an open cholecystectomy, a patient can remain in hospital after the surgery for up to 5 days with the recovery period being anything between six and eight weeks.

As with any form of surgery, it is advisable to take it easy with anything that could put strain on your back or the incision point until you feel better. The good thing about the human body is that it is able to communicate when it is in a position to do or not do something. With that said, pay attention to what your body is telling you.

Possible side effects of a gallbladder removal surgery

Patients can live a perfectly normal life after their gallbladder has been removed and so most of the side effects usually dissipate with time.

Some of the short term side effects include:

- Lethargy – this can be as a result of the heavy painkillers administered after the surgery or the anesthesia, which usually pass within a day.

- Bruised, painful and swollen wounds – these will fade away with a few days and the pain killers prescribed usually help take away the discomfort.

- Diarrhea, gas and bloating – this can last for up to 2 months. Eating foods that are high in fiber (both soluble and insoluble) such as veggies, fruit and whole grains can help make your stool firm. However, your doctor may also prescribe some drugs depending on the severity of your symptoms.

- Irritability, fatigue and mood swings - these often occur as a result of your body showing frustration of the reduced motor skills. However, as you recover, you will notice these symptoms also disappearing.

- Pain in shoulders and stomach – this is the side effect of the gas used to inflate your stomach during the surgery and will pass within a couple of days. Prescribed painkillers will help reduce the discomfort.

Taking care of the wounds

Dissolvable stitches are most commonly used to close up the wounds after surgery. You should notice the stitches beginning to disappear within the first 2 weeks.

However, if your surgeon used the non-dissolvable stitches, you will need to go back to the hospital to get them removed after 1 week or 10 days, depending on what your doctor tells you.

Before you leave the hospital, ensure a nurse or your doctor shows you how to look after the wounds and stitches including how often you need to change the dressings and when you can take a bath or shower.

If you no one to assist you at home, you may want to have a nurse come over and help you to avoid the risk of infection.

Eating After Your Cholecystectomy

Most people who have their gallbladder removed are people who have had a painful and arduous journey with gall stones. If you are in this category, then you know that fatty foods are a huge no no as they can exacerbate the pain. Having a cholecystectomy takes away that problem. However, after your surgery, you may experience some digestive problems as your digestive system adjusts to the new norm.

It is important that you understand that the gallbladder is not necessary for proper digestion of the food you eat but you also need to give your body time to adjust to your cholecystectomy. You may experience bloating and diarrhea when you eat fatty foods up to one month after having your surgery.

To reduce and even eliminate digestive discomfort, here are some practical and healthy tips:

- Don't go ham!

Now that you don't have to worry about painful gallstones doesn't mean you should go ham on all the foods that you love but couldn't eat prior to your surgery. Remember, a member of your digestive tract has just been removed and as such you need to give your body time to adjust. The best thing you can do is to ease into food. Actually, within the first weeks you should eat the same diet your doctor recommended when you had to deal with gallstones. Then as you recover better from your wound and as your body adjusts to not having a gallbladder start easing into some of the fatty foods. The key being healthy! Right after surgery, depending on what type of surgery (keyhole or open) you had, your doctor may recommend very soft or liquid foods or let you eat what you desire. To avoid uncomfortable digestive consequences, you should stick to soft and bland foods such as white rice, bananas, boiled potatoes, dry bread and plain pasta as these are easy to digest.

As you heal, you will be able to add variety to your diet with our meal plan providing you with delicious, healthy and easy recipes.

- Approach dairy with caution

Dairy foods are an amazing natural source of vitamin D, calcium and protein. However, after a cholecystectomy, full fat dairy products can cause painful bloating and even diarrhea. To be safe, only eat low fat options such as cheeses and skim milk. Taking low-fat yogurt can actually help with digestion due to its probiotic content that helps aid digestion.

As you heal, you can slowly start introducing full-fat dairy products.

- Drink plenty of water

If you are experiencing diarrhea after your surgery, you need to take in a lot of water to help re-hydrate your body from all the lost fluids. You can enhance your water with vitamins and you can also ask your doctor to recommend a beverage that will help increase your electrolyte intake. Stay away from caffeinated drinks such as energy drinks, coffee and tea.

Even after the diarrhea wanes, continue taking plenty of water, at least 8 glasses of water each day, in order as this will help improve your digestion and also keep your cells healthy.

- Steadily increase your fiber intake

Fiber intake after a gallbladder removal surgery is like a double edged sword. On one hand it will help bulk up your stool thus stopping diarrhea but on the other hand it can worsen bloating and flatulence.

To have smoother transition after your surgery, you should introduce fiber into your diet very slowly. In the beginning, start only by taking fruit and veggie juices that have no fiber then little by little start taking blended juices that have some fiber then move into taking actual fruit, veggies and other high fiber foods such as brown rice, legumes, nuts and cereals.

- Healthy low fat foods

A short period after your gallbladder removal surgery, your body is going to face challenges digesting fat. This is because you have mostly stayed for such a long time without eating fat. Your body therefore has to remind itself how to deal with fats in the digestive tract. This can lead to diarrhea and bloating in the initial phase.

It is therefore advisable to stick to low-fat foods in the period right after your surgery and gradually increase the amount of healthy fatty foods you eat as you recover. For a start eat lean foods such as skinless white meat, baked fish and turkey breast.

Once you've recovered, the doctor should give you a go head, you can now gradually add fats to your diet. It's okay to indulge here and there in some of the foods you could never eat before. However, the goal is to stay healthy so ultimately focus on healthy foods.

Focus on developing a healthy lifestyle

For most people who have had their gallbladders removed, healing from the surgery is akin to a license to indulge in all the foods they couldn't eat before such as pizza, fries, burgers and other fatty fast food. while your body is now in a position to handle fat, throwing all caution to the wind when it comes to the food we eat can have a lot of adverse effects such as obesity, developing heart problems, diabetes, to mention but a few.

The goal in life is to live a happy, healthy and fulfilled life. You will look and feel like the food you eat; this is a general rule of thumb. If you focus on junk food that is doused in sugar, fats, salt and artificial additives, your health will be a mirror reflection of that. If on the other hand you eat clean, healthy and natural food and go an extra step of exercising on a regular basis, at least 30 minutes every day, you are going to be the perfect picture of health and you will be surprised at how much younger you are going to look.

Getting a cholecystectomy is like getting a new lease of life. Do your best to take good care of your body by nourishing it with foods that actually support the functionality of every single organ in your body and you are going to enjoy living life.

Our recipe section does an amazing job of guiding you on how you should be eating for the rest of your life. Tasty, healthy, super simple and creative, you are going to love making our featured dishes. Once you get a great hang of it, feel free to modify the recipes to your customized taste and to also create new recipes for yourself getting inspiration from what we have done already.

Healthy No Gallbladder Food List

Once you are fully recovered, you are now free to eat any type of food unless you already have a pre-existing condition such as diabetes that doesn't allow you to eat some foods. Something important to consider when deciding on what foods you are going to be consuming and that are now going to become a regular part of your pantry is the goal you have in mind for your body and health.

For example, if you are trying to lose weight, you shouldn't be consuming foods that are very high in carbs and even when it comes to the carbs you should be taking, they should be complex unprocessed carbs.

In this section, we are going to look at a healthy food list that will help you stay healthy and make delicious food like what we have in our recipe section.

Healthy fats and oils

Olive oil is healthy for your heart and overall functioning of your body as it's a great source of unsaturated fats that help lower your bad cholesterol levels thus keeping your heart healthy. Go for extra virgin olive oil and when cooking use a small flame and don't let it burn as this denatures it. Other healthy fats and oil sources include avocadoes, coconuts, nuts and fatty fish such as wild caught salmon.

Vegetables and Fruits

Fruits and veggies are endowed with vitamins, fiber, protein, minerals and potent plant compounds that fight off disease causing free radicals. Add cranberries, avocadoes, grapes, beets, berries, oranges, bell peppers, broccoli, kale, watercress, radishes, fennel, and cauliflower. Basically, if it's a fruit or veggie and is endowed with healthy nutrients, then it should be part of your diet.

When it comes to fruits and veggies, your choice is going to be based on whether you are following any diet. For example, if you are on a keto diet, you know that your fruit intake is very limited as it eliminates all fruits that are high in carbs. The same thing for vegetables.

If you have a pre-existing condition, you will also choose fruits and veggies that your doctor has advised should be part of your diet and eliminate the rest.

Poultry, Fish and Meat

Poultry, fish and meat are great sources of protein for your body. When buying these, be keen to go for lean cuts only but for fish, you can enjoy fatty fish as they contain omega-3 fatty acids that are actually good for your overall health. It is also important that you avoid processed meats that have very high sodium levels.

Whenever possible, you should opt for free range poultry, grass fed meats and wild caught fish as they do not have any hormonal residues from the food and medication administered to the animals before slaughter.

Whole Grains

Whole grains are an amazing source of fiber, complex carbs, folate and minerals that aid the digestion process. Some healthy options of whole grains include; brown rice, bran cereal, oats and legumes. Avoid processed grains as these have been stripped off their fiber content and some of their mineral content as well leaving you with high calorie foods that are devoid of any nutrition.

Water is your best beverage

Your body needs to stay hydrated in order to operate at peak performance in all of its functions. Water helps flush out toxins which can help the liver not get overburdened by the detoxification process. It also helps your digestive system optimally digest the food you have taken and it helps your cells rejuvenate leaving you looking young and healthy.

Take caffeine and alcohol moderately

While your gallbladder has been removed and you can take all the caffeine and alcohol you can, it is wise to take care of your body and keep it healthy. You do this by reducing the amount of caffeine or alcohol that you consume. There is one thing you are going to notice after partaking our 30 day meal plan no gallbladder program: your elevated energy levels. When you provide your body with clean and healthy nutrition and take the initiative to stay limber by exercising on a regular basis, you will not have any need for a pick me up in the form of caffeine because you don't have any natural energy left.

The body was designed to e fully functional by itself and the only thing it requires from you is for you to provide it with clean fuel. Enjoy an occasional indulgence of alcohol but don't let it be your regular habit. Service your body well and it is going to provide you with great and long service without you having to worry about a particular organ not working properly because you will make it your personal goal to properly nourish your body.

Go nuts, but in moderation

Now that you don't have to worry about significantly keeping your fat intake level to an absolute minimum, you can go ahead and enjoy the great variety of nuts. However, it is essential to eat nuts in moderation as eating too many nuts may increase your fat intake which can be a problem if you are on a weight loss journey.

Additionally, nuts have healthy fat and fiber along with plant sterols. Plant sterols when taken in excess can block the absorption of cholesterol in your body. Moderation is therefore key. You can consume nuts as snacks or sprinkle them on salads, cereals and meat dishes and soups.

Increase your consumption of plant-based Foods

A healthy diet offers several nutrients to your body. You will get antioxidants, minerals, vitamins and fiber from plant-based foods. Antioxidants help your body fight of free radicals and also eliminate toxins.

Your body can develop free radicals because of environmental stresses and natural processes, such as processed foods. The build-up of free radicals may increase the chances of oxidative stress. It can increase the chances of cell damage that will be the reason for cancer, premature aging and several other diseases.

Healthy minerals found in natural foods

There are so many vital minerals that our bodies need for proper functioning that can only be found in the food we eat. Calcium, for example is available in broccoli, kale, and other leafy, dark greens. Moreover, it is available in milk, cheese, and yogurt. Some fortified alternatives to dairy are nut milk such almond milk.

Other vitamins and minerals essential to your health are magnesium, phosphorus, vitamin C. Fresh vegetables and fruits offer these nutrients. You can find vitamin C in citrus foods, oranges, green and red peppers, broccoli, kiwifruit, tomatoes, and strawberries.

Magnesium rich foods include cashews, almonds, peanut butter, peanuts, beans, spinach, edamame, potato, soy milk, rice, avocado, banana and yogurt. Excellent sources of folate are beef liver, black-eyed peas, spinach, fortified cereals, and asparagus. While you can get these minerals from supplements, it is always better to get them from fresh dietary sources unless prescribed by your doctor.

30-DAY GALLBLADDER SURGERY DIET MEAL PLAN

Make sure that the calories intake is sufficient for your body.

Day	Breakfast	AM SNACK	Lunch	PM SNACK	Dinner
DAY 1	Oil-Free Lemon & Avocado Pancakes	Toasted Almonds & Seed Mix	Avocado & Cucumber Salad with Toasted Nuts and Seeds	Handful Blueberries	Grilled Chicken Breast with Nutty Pesto
DAY 2	Crunchy Breakfast Porridge with Toasted Coconut	1 Green Apple	Delicious Green Soup with Brown Rice	Creamy Lemon Corn Snack	Grilled Salmon with Creamy Salsa
DAY 3	Healthy Guacamole with Whole-Wheat Bread	Turmeric Nut & Coconut Balls	Avocado & Mixed Veggie Salad with Garlic Vinaigrette	1 Pear	Chicken Cacciatore with Brown Rice
DAY 4	Creamy Avocado Breakfast Smoothie	1 Grapefruit	Citrusy Soup with Caramelized Onions	Dried Fruit & Nut Mix	Lemony Salmon with Crunchy Slaw
DAY 5	Lemon and Blueberry Oil-Free Pancakes	Healthy Berry & Nut Bars	Healthy Superfood Salad with Lemon-Tahini Dressing	Handful Blueberries	Turkey Patty Salad with Lemony Tahini Sauce
DAY 6	Crunchy Breakfast Muesli	1 Banana	Lemon-Coconut Stir-Fried Greens	Tangy Carrot & Parsnips French Fries	Tasty Lemon Salmon Bake
DAY 7	Shrimp Omelet with Salsa	Vinegar & Salt Kale Chips	Super Healthy Salad with Lemony Dressing	1 Pear	Delicious Mung & Veggie Stew with Avocado

DAY 8	Avocado & Spirulina Chia Pudding	1 Green Apple	Stir-Fried Tofu and Veggies	Roasted Chickpea	Prawns Served with Whole-Wheat Bread
DAY 9		Healthy Guacamole	Crunchy Rainbow Detox Salad	1 Grapefruit	Crunchy Fried Tofu with Greens
DAY 10	Creamy Grapefruit & Blackberry Smoothie Bowl	Handful Grapes	Crunchy Vegetable Sauté	Healthy Raw Bars	Coconut & Lemon Chicken Bake
DAY 11	Oil-Free Coconut Buckwheat Pancakes with Orange Juice	Toasted Almonds & Seed Mix	Crunchy Superfood Cleanse Salad	1 Pear	Stir-Fried Veggies with Seared Lemon Chicken
DAY 12	Healthy Overnight Oats	Handful Blueberries	Black Bean Soup	Tahini Dip	Grilled Burritos with Cashew Crema
DAY 13	Healthy Green Acai Bowl	Avocado & Pea Dip with Carrots	Healthy Vegetable Salad	1 Green Apple	Scrumptious Ratatouille
DAY 14	Buckwheat Breakfast Cereal	1 Pear	Chicken & Zucchini Soup	Healthy Superfood Raw Bars	Lemon Grilled Fish with Salsa
DAY 15	Healthy Breakfast Porridge	Apricot-Sesame Balls	Crunchy Steak Salad	1 Orange	Superfood Toasted Almonds Wraps
DAY 16	Pineapple & Ginger Breakfast Smoothie	1 Pear	Healthy Lentil Soup	Turmeric Nut & Coconut Balls	Spiced Lentils with Brown Rice
DAY 17	Healthy Tofu Scramble	Almond Coconut Protein Bars	Super Cleansing Lunch Salad	1 Grapefruit	Healthy Chickpea Veggie Sauté

DAY 18	Healthy Breakfast Muesli	Handful Grapes	Lunch Turkey Lettuce Wraps	Roasted Pumpkin Seeds	Mushroom Marinara with Buckwheat Pasta
DAY 19	Mushroom and Veggie Omelets	Whole Grain Crackers	Sweet Beet Salad with Toasted Pumpkin Seeds	1 Green Apple	Chicken Cacciatore with Brown Rice
DAY 20	Healthy Green Smoothie	Handful Blueberries	Stir-Fried Chicken & Veggies	Raw Banana Mash Snack	Tasty Lemon Salmon Bake
DAY 21	Fish Breakfast Frittata	Roasted Pumpkin Seeds	Veggie Salad with Toasted Pumpkin Seeds	1 Pear	BBQ Chicken Breast Salad
DAY 22	Lemon and Blueberry Oil-Free Pancakes	1 Grapefruit	Mushroom & Buckwheat Dish	Berry Power Bars	Delicious Sweet Potato & Bean Curry
DAY 23	Mushroom and Veggie Omelets	Dried Fruit & Nut Mix	Sweet Potato & Scallion Salad	1 Green Apple	Stir-Fried Chicken & Green Bean
DAY 24	Oil-Free Coconut Buckwheat Pancakes with Orange Juice	Handful Grapes	Millet Stir Fry with Veggies	Tangy Carrot & Parsnips French Fries	Veggie Noodles in Coconut Sauce
DAY 25	Pineapple & Ginger Breakfast Smoothie	Healthy Superfood Raw Bars	Avocado, Cucumber & Tomato Salad	Handful Blueberries	Lime Turkey Breast & Avocado Salad
DAY 26	Healthy Guacamole with Whole-Wheat Bread	1 Grapefruit	Delicious Turkey Soup	Toasted Almonds & Seed Mix	Prawns Served with Whole-Wheat Bread

DAY 27	Healthy Breakfast Shake	Apricot-Sesame Balls	Cleansing Superfood Salad	1 Pear	Stir-Fried Veggies with Seared Lemon Chicken
DAY 28	Oil-Free Lemon & Avocado Pancakes	1 Orange	Lunch Millet Lettuce Wraps	Avocado & Pea Dip with Carrots	Grilled Chicken Breast with Nutty Greek Yogurt
DAY 29	Crunchy Breakfast Muesli	Creamy Lemon Corn Snack	Avocado & Cucumber Salad with Toasted Nuts and Seeds	1 Green Apple	Pan-Seared Turkey with Orange Chimichurri
DAY 30	Crunchy Breakfast Porridge with Toasted Coconut	Handful Blueberries	Citrusy Soup with Caramelized Onions	Healthy Berry & Nut Bars	Lemon Grilled Fish with Salsa

HEALTHY GALLBLADDER SURGERY DIET BREAKFAST RECIPES

1. Creamy Avocado Breakfast Smoothie

Yield: 3 Servings
Total Time: 10 Minutes
Prep Time: 10 Minutes
Cook Time: N/A

Ingredients

- o 3 cups unsweetened almond milk
- o 1 avocado, diced
- o 1 tablespoon ground flaxseed
- o 1 tablespoon almond butter
- o 1 teaspoon minced fresh ginger
- o 2 cups chopped spinach
- o 1 cup frozen blueberries
- o 2 tablespoons toasted coconut flakes
- o 2 tablespoons raw honey

Directions

Combine all ingredients in a blender and blend until very smooth and creamy.
Divide the smoothie between serving bowls and top each with more blueberries and coconut flakes. Enjoy!

Nutrition information per Serving:

Calories: 350; Total Fat: 22.4 g; Net Carbs: 22.1 g; Dietary Fiber: 8.7 g; Sugars: 17.6 g; Protein: 4.4 g; Cholesterol: 0 mg; Sodium: 222 mg

2. Crunchy Breakfast Porridge with Toasted Coconut

Yield: 1 Serving
Total Time: 7 Minutes
Prep Time: 5 Minutes
Cook Time: 2 Minutes

Ingredients

- 1 cup unsweetened almond milk
- 2 tablespoons ground flaxseeds
- 1/2 cup almond flour
- 1 tablespoon coconut oil
- 1 teaspoon cinnamon
- ¼ teaspoon sea salt
- 1 cup water
- 1 teaspoon raw honey
- 2 tablespoons toasted coconut
- 2 tablespoons toasted almonds

Directions

In a microwave safe bowl, stir together all the ingredients until well combined; place in the microwave and heat for 1 minute.

Stir again to mix well and microwave for another 1 minute. Serve right away topped with toasted almonds and toasted coconut.

Nutritional Information per Serving:

Calories: 694; Total Fat: 57.4 g; Net Carbs: 15.2 g; Dietary Fiber: 14.4 g; Sugars: 7.2 g; Protein: 18.6 g; Cholesterol: 0 mg; Sodium: 782 mg

3. Oil-FreeLemon &Avocado Pancakes

Yield: 3 Servings
Total Time: 20 Minutes
Prep Time: 10 Minutes
Cook Time: 10 Minutes

Ingredients

- 1 ripe avocado
- 1 1/4 cups almond flour
- 1/2 cup fresh lemon juice
- 1/2 cup unsweetened almond milk
- 1 teaspoon raw honey
- 1 tablespoon baking powder
- 1 teaspoon matcha powder
- 1 teaspoon vanilla extract
- Pinch of salt
- 1 cup fresh blueberries to serve

Directions

In a blender, blend together all ingredients until smooth.

Heat a nonstick skillet over medium heat; add in batter and spread into a circle.

Cook for about 2 minutes per side or until browned. Repeat with the remaining batter.

Serve topped with fresh blueberries.

Enjoy!

Nutritional Information per Serving:

Calories: 478; Total Fat: 36.3 g; Net Carbs: 16.8 g; Dietary Fiber: 11.5 g; Sugars: 8.2 g; Protein: 12.5 g; Cholesterol: 0 mg; Sodium: 115 mg

4. Healthy Guacamole with Whole-Wheat Bread

Yield: 6 Servings
Total Time: 10 Minutes
Prep Time: 10 Minutes
Cook Time: 0 Minutes

Ingredients

- 2 medium avocadoes
- 1 tablespoon chopped sun-dried tomatoes
- 6 cherry tomatoes, halved
- 2 tablespoons freshly squeezed lemon juice
- 1 red onion, finely chopped
- A handful of freshly chopped parsley
- 1 teaspoon fresh oregano, chopped
- ½ teaspoon sea salt
- ½ teaspoon black pepper
- 6 slices of whole-wheat bread

Directions

Cut the avocadoes in half and remove the seed. Scoop out the flesh into a large bowl and use a fork to mash it up to desired consistency.

Sprinkle the lemon juice on the mashed avocado and mx well until well combined. Add in all the remaining ingredients and mix well until well incorporated.

Adjust the salt, pepper and herbs, if need be. If you like your guacamole tangier, squeeze in more lemon juice and for a more tomatoey flavor, add the sun-dried tomatoes.

Serve immediately with whole multi-grain bread.

Enjoy!

Nutritional Information per Serving:

Calories: 245; Total Fat: 14.8 g; Net Carbs: 16.2 g; Dietary Fiber: 8.9 g; Sugars: 6.2 g; Protein: 6.6 g; Cholesterol: 0 mg; Sodium: 331 mg

5. Crunchy Breakfast Muesli

Yield: 6 Servings
Total Time: 5 Minutes
Prep Time: 5 Minutes
Cook Time: N/A

Ingredients

- 3 cups unsweetened almond milk (or cashew milk)
- 1 cup hemp seeds
- 1/2 cup chia seeds
- 1 cup sunflower seeds
- 1 cup pumpkin seeds
- 1/4 cup dried apricot
- 1/4 cup dried cranberries
- 1/2 cup unsweetened toasted coconut flakes
- 1/4 cup fresh strawberries
- 1/4 cup fresh blueberries
- 1/4 cup fresh raspberries
- 1 apple, diced

Directions

Mix seeds, dry fruit and toasted coconut flakes in a large bowl; stir in milk until well combined and then serve topped with berries and diced apple.

Nutritional Information per Serving:

Calories: 471; Total Fat: 34.5 g; Net Carbs: 16.2 g; Dietary Fiber: 11 g; Sugars: 7.1 g; Protein: 17.9 g; Cholesterol: 0 mg; Sodium: 114 mg

6. Avocado &Spirulina Chia Pudding

Yield: 3 Servings
Total Time: 35 Minutes
Prep Time: 10 Minutes
Cook Time: N/A

Ingredients

- 4 tablespoons chia seeds
- 3 cups unsweetened almond milk
- 2 teaspoons raw honey
- 2 tablespoons spirulina powder
- 1 avocado, diced
- 1 ripe banana
- 2 cups blueberries
- 2 tablespoons toasted coconut flakes
- 2 tablespoons chopped toasted cashews

Directions

In a bowl, mix together half of the almond milk, maple syrup and chia seeds; let sit for at least 30 minutes or until all liquid is absorbed.

In a food processor, blend together the remaining almond milk, blueberries, spirulina, banana, and avocado until very smooth.

Divide the chia seed mixture into serving bowls and top each serving with a layer of spirulina puree. Serve topped with toasted coconut flakes, chia seeds, and toasted cashews.

Nutritional Information per Serving:

Calories: 406; Total Fat: 25.4 g; Net Carbs: 14.4 g; Dietary Fiber: 28.4 g; Sugars: 39.2 g; Protein: 9.4 g; Cholesterol: 0 mg; Sodium: 240 mg

7. Creamy Grapefruit & Blackberry Smoothie Bowl

Yield: 2 Servings
Total Time: 5 Minutes
Prep Time: 5 Minutes
Cook Time: N/A

Ingredients

- 2 cups fresh blackberries
- 2 cups fresh spinach
- 2 cups unsweetened almond milk
- 1 grapefruit, peeled, segmented
- 1 cup fresh lemon juice
- 1 avocado
- 2 tablespoons chia seeds
- 2 tablespoons toasted pumpkin seeds
- ½ cup toasted coconut flakes
- ½ cup toasted chopped almonds

Directions

In a blender, blend together blackberry, almond milk, avocado, lemon juice, grapefruit, and spinach until very smooth and creamy; add in blackberries and pulse to combine well. Divide the smooth among serving bowls and top each serving with fresh toasted almonds, pumpkin seeds, toasted coconut flakes, and chia seeds.
Enjoy!

Nutritional Information per Serving:

Calories: 668; Total Fat: 50.6 g; Net Carbs: 21.4 g; Dietary Fiber: 25.8 g; Sugars: 17 g; Protein: 16.6 g; Cholesterol: 0 mg; Sodium: 244 mg

8. Lemon and Blueberry Oil-Free Pancakes

Servings: 8 Pancakes (4 Servings)
Total Time: 20 Minutes
Prep Time: 10 Minutes
Cook Time: 10 Minutes

Ingredients

- 1 cup almond flour
- 1/4 cup coconut flour
- 1 cup unsweetened almond milk
- 1/4 cup fresh lemon juice
- 2 free-range eggs
- 1 cup blueberries
- 1 tablespoon fresh lemon zest
- 1 tablespoon raw honey
- 1 teaspoon vanilla extract
- 1 teaspoon baking soda

Directions

In a large bowl, whisk together eggs, vanilla, raw honey and lemon zest until well combined; whisk in coconut flour until well blended. Whisk in almond flour, baking soda, and lemon juice until very smooth.

Heat a nonstick skillet over medium heat; add in two spoonfuls on batter and spread into a circle. Cook for about 2 minutes per side and then repeat with the remaining ingredients. Divide the fresh blueberries among the pancakes and fold to make wraps. Serve warm.

Enjoy!

Nutritional Information per Serving:

Calories: 308; Total Fat: 20.3 g; Net Carbs: 14.6 g; Dietary Fiber: 7.2 g; Sugars: 8.6 g; Protein: 10.4 g; Cholesterol: 82 mg; Sodium: 382 mg

9. Healthy Breakfast Shake

Yield: 4 Servings
Total Time: 5 Minutes
Prep Time: 5 Minutes
Cook Time: N/A

Ingredients

- 1 cup blackberries
- 1 cup blueberries
- 1 cup raspberries
- 2 cups unsweetened almond milk
- 1 avocado
- 1 teaspoon cinnamon
- 1 tablespoon raw honey
- 4 tablespoons almond butter

Directions

Blend everything together until very smooth. Enjoy!

Nutritional Information per Serving:

Calories: 290; Total Fat: 21.1 g; Net Carbs: 14.9 g; Dietary Fiber: 10.6 g; Sugars: 12 g; Protein: 6 g; Cholesterol: 0 mg; Sodium: 95 mg

10.   Shrimp Omelet with Salsa

Yields: 3 Servings
Total Time: 40 Minutes
Prep Time: 10 Minutes
Cook Time: 30 Minutes

Ingredients

- 200g shrimp, peeled and de-veined
- 1 red onion, chopped
- 2 cloves garlic, minced
- 6 large free-range eggs, beaten
- 2 tablespoons fresh lemon juice
- 1 medium avocado, diced
- 2 medium tomatoes, diced
- 3 spring onions, chopped
- 1 tablespoon coconut oil
- 1/8 teaspoon black pepper
- 1/4 teaspoon sea salt
- 1 tablespoon chopped cilantro

Directions

Cook shrimp in a skillet set over medium heat until it turns pink; chop the cooked shrimp and set aside.

In a small bowl, toss together fresh lemon juice, avocado, tomato, spring onions, and cilantro; season with sea salt and pepper and set aside.

In a separate bowl, beat the eggs and set aside.

Set a skillet over medium heat; add coconut oil and heat until hot. Sauté half of red onion and garlic until fragrant.

Add half of the egg to the skillet and tilt the skillet to cover the bottom. When almost cooked, add half of the shrimp onto one side of the egg and fold in half. Cook for 1 minute more and transfer to a plate.

Repeat with the remaining ingredients for the second omelet. Serve the shrimp omelet topped with the avocado-tomato mixture. Enjoy!

Nutritional Information Per Serving:

Calories: 434; Total Fat: 30.8 g; Net Carbs: 8.6 g; Dietary Fiber: 6.4 g; Sugars: 5.1 g; Protein: 30.4 g; Cholesterol: 384 mg; Sodium: 353 mg

11.   Healthy Overnight Oats

Yield: 2 Servings
Total Time: 10 Minutes + Chilling Time
Prep Time: 10 Minutes
Cook Time: N/A

Ingredients

- 1/2 cup old-fashioned oats
- 1 teaspoon chia seeds
- 1/2 cup vanilla almond milk (unsweetened)
- 1/4 cup fresh blueberries
- 1/4 banana, chopped
- 1/4 cup chopped fresh pineapple
- 1/4 teaspoon cinnamon
- 1 tablespoon chopped toasted almonds

Directions

In a small jar, combine oats, chia seeds, almond milk, blueberries, banana, pineapple, yogurt, cinnamon and chopped toasted almonds. Refrigerate overnight.
To serve, remove from the fridge and stir to mix well before serving.

Nutritional Information per Serving:

Calories: 310; Total Fat: 18.4 g; Net Carbs: 24 g; Dietary Fiber: 5 g; Sugars: 10.2 g
Protein: 10.8 g; Cholesterol: 3 mg; Sodium: 29 mg

12. Buckwheat Breakfast Cereal

Yield: 4 Servings
Total Time: 55 Minutes
Prep Time: 15 Minutes
Cook Time: 40 Minutes

Ingredients

- 1 cup buckwheat groats
- 1 tablespoon olive oil, or to taste
- 1 red onion, diced
- 1 carrot, diced
- ½ pound mushrooms, diced
- 1 tablespoon coconut oil
- 2 cups water
- A pinch of sea salt
- A pinch of black pepper

Directions

Rinse buckwheat and drain.

Heat a nonstick skillet over medium heat and cook in buckwheat for about 5 minutes or until toasted; transfer to a large bowl and set aside.

Add olive oil to the skillet and cook in onions and carrots for about 10 minutes or until tender; stir in mushrooms and cook for about 5 minutes.

In a pot set over medium heat, melt coconut oil and stir in buckwheat; add in the onion mixture, salt, pepper and water and bring a gentle boil. Simmer for about 20 minutes and then serve right away.

Nutritional Information per Serving:

Calories: 185; Total Fat: 7.5 g; Net Carbs: 22.6 g; Dietary Fiber: 4.5 g; Sugars: 3.7 g
Protein: 6 g; Cholesterol: 8 mg; Sodium: 101 mg

13.   Oil-Free Coconut Buckwheat Pancakes with Orange Juice

Yield: 5 Servings
Total Time: 35 Minutes
Prep Time: 15 Minutes
Cook Time: 20 Minutes

Ingredients

- 1 cup buckwheat groats
- 1 ½ cups boiling water
- 1 cup spelt flour
- ½ cup shredded coconut
- 2 teaspoons baking powder
- 1 cup low fat milk
- 1 egg
- 1 teaspoon raw honey
- 1 serving cooking spray

Directions

Combine buckwheat and boiling water in a large bowl and let sit for at least 10 minutes or until water is absorbed.

Heat a nonstick skillet over medium heat.

In another bowl, whisk together buckwheat, coconut, flour, and baking powder.

In a small bowl, whisk together oil, egg, milk and raw honey; pour into the buckwheat mixture and wheat to blend well.

Heat a nonstick skillet and add in about a third cup of the batter, spreading to cover the bottom.

Cook for about 2 minutes per side or until the pancakes are golden browned.

Repeat with the remaining batter.

Serve the pancakes with a glass of fresh orange juice.

Nutritional Information per Serving:

Calories: 297; Total Fat: 11.7 g; Net Carbs: 36.8 g; Dietary Fiber: 6.1 g; Sugars: 6.8 g Protein: 9.8 g; Cholesterol: 33 mg; Sodium: 69 mg

14.   Pineapple & Ginger Breakfast Smoothie

Serving Total: 3 servings
Total Time: 5Minutes
Prep Time: 5 Minutes
Cook Time: 0 Minutes

Ingredients
- o   1 cup pineapple chunks
- o   1-inch fresh ginger root, peeled
- o   1-inh fresh turmeric root, peeled
- o   1/2 cup fresh lemon juice
- o   1 teaspoon raw honey
- o   1 tablespoon almond butter
- o   1 cup coconut water

Directions
Combine all the ingredients in your blender and pulse until smooth.
Serve in a tall glass.
Enjoy!

Nutritional Information per Serving:
Calories: 111; Total Fat: 3.7 g; Carbs: 18.7 g; Dietary Fiber 2.5 g; Sugars: 14.4 g; Protein: 2.4 g; Cholesterol: 0 mg; Sodium: 94 mg

15.   Healthy Breakfast Muesli

Yield: 6 Servings
Total Time: 20 Minutes
Prep Time: 20 Minutes
Cook Time: N/A

Ingredients

- 1 cup quinoa
- 1 cup wheat flakes
- 2 cups old fashioned oats
- 1/2 cup walnuts
- 1/2 cup raw pumpkin seeds
- 1/2 cup sliced almonds
- 1/2 cup ground flax seeds
- 1/2 cup hemp hearts
- 1/2 cup raisins
- 1/2 cup coconut flakes
- 1 teaspoon Almond extract
- 1 teaspoon cinnamon
- 4 cups almond milk, to serve
- Berries, to serve

Directions

Stir together all the ingredients in a large bowl. Serve with almond milk and berries.

Nutritional Information per Serving:

Calories: 625 Total Fat: 26.5 g; Carbs: 77.9 g; Dietary Fiber: 13.6 g; Sugars: 10.3 g; Protein: 20.9 g; Cholesterol: 0 mg; Sodium: 39 mg

16. Healthy Green Smoothie

Yield: 2 Servings
Total Time: 5 Minutes
Prep Time: 5 Minutes
Cook Time: N/A

Ingredients

- 1 cup unsweetened almond milk
- 1 frozen banana
- 2 cups baby spinach
- 2tablespoons natural almond butter
- 1/8 teaspoon ground nutmeg
- 1/4 teaspoon ground cinnamon
- 1/2 teaspoon ground ginger
- 1 scoop vanilla protein powder
- 1/2 teaspoon vanilla extract

Directions

Blend together all the ingredients until very smooth. Serve topped with cinnamon and hemp seeds. Enjoy!

Nutritional Information per Serving:

Calories: 199 Total Fat: 7.9 g; Carbs: 19 g; Dietary Fiber: 3.8 g; Sugars: 8.9 g; Protein: 15.8 g; Cholesterol: 15 mg; Sodium: 39 mg

17.   Mushroom and Veggie Omelets

Yield: 2 Servings
Total Time: 25 Minutes
Prep Time: 10 Minutes
Cook Time: 15 Minutes

Ingredients

- 3 egg whites
- 1 egg
- 1/2 teaspoon extra-virgin olive oil
- 1/8 teaspoon garlic powder
- A pinch of salt
- 1/2 cup sliced cremini mushrooms
- 2 tablespoons chopped red bell pepper
- 1/4 cup chopped green onion
- 1 cup chopped fresh kale

Directions

In a large bowl, whisk together egg whites, egg, garlic powder, nutmeg, and salt until well blended.

Heat olive oil in a skillet over medium heat; add green onion, mushrooms and belle pepper and cook for about 5 minutes or until tender.

Stir in egg mixture and cook for about 5 minutes per side or until egg is set. Slice and serve hot.

Nutrition information per Serving:

Calories: 133; Total Fat: 3.9 g; Carbs: 15 g; Dietary Fiber: 2.7 g; Sugars: 7.2 g; Protein: 11.1 g; Cholesterol: 82 mg; Sodium: 179 mg

18.   Healthy Green Acai Bowl

Yield: 2 Servings
Total Time: 10 Minutes
Prep Time: 10 Minutes
Cook Time: N/A

Ingredients

- ½ cup blackberries
- ½ cup strawberries
- ½ cup raspberries
- 1 heaped tablespoon acai powder
- 1 cup chopped kale leaves
- 1 cup unsweetened almond milk
- 1/2 cup sliced berries for topping

Directions

In a blender, blend all ingredients until very smooth. Sprinkle with and sliced berries and serve.

Nutritional Information per Serving:

Calories: 99; Total Fat: 2.2 g; Carbs: 18.7 g; Dietary Fiber: 6.6 g; Sugars: 7.4 g; Protein: 2.6 g; Cholesterol: 0 mg; Sodium: 63 mg

19.   HealthyBreakfast Porridge

Yield: 1 Serving
Total Time: 10 Minutes
Prep Time: 10 Minutes
Cook Time: 10 Minutes

Ingredients

- ¼ cup unsweetened almond milk
- 1 tablespoon chopped almonds or walnuts
- 1 teaspoon ground flaxseed
- 1 tablespoon chia seeds
- 1 tablespoon shredded unsweetened coconut
- 1 teaspoon pure vanilla extract

Toppings:

- 1 teaspoon peanut butter
- 1 teaspoon toasted coconut

Directions

In a large bowl, mix all ingredients together; refrigerate, covered, overnight. Divide porridge into serving bowls and top with peanut butter, and toasted coconut.

Nutritional Information per Serving:

Calories: 287; Total Fat: 20.9 g; Carbs: 17 g; Dietary Fiber: 12.4 g; Sugars: 1.8 g; Protein: 8.9 g; Cholesterol: 0 mg; Sodium: 77 mg

20.   Healthy Tofu Scramble

Yield: 3 Servings
Total Time: 35 Minutes
Prep Time: 20 Minutes
Cook Time: 15 Minutes

Ingredients
- o   1 pound extra firm tofu, drained and pressed
- o   1 1/2 cups mushrooms, sliced
- o   1/4 of an onion, diced
- o   1/2 cup halved cherry tomatoes
- o   1 garlic clove, minced
- o   2 teaspoons fresh parsley
- o   1/2 teaspoon dry mustard
- o   1/4 teaspoon turmeric
- o   1/2 teaspoon sea salt

Directions
Heat a tablespoon of oil in a skillet set over medium heat; sauté garlic and onion for about 2 minutes or until fragrant. Stir in mushrooms and cook for about 5 minutes or until lightly browned.

Crumble in tofu and stir in turmeric, mustard, and salt; cook for about 5 minutes or until heated through. Remove from heat and stir in tomatoes. Serve hot!

Nutritional Information per Serving:
Calories: 95; Total Fat: 5.1 g; Carbs: 4.5 g; Dietary Fiber: 1.8 g; Sugars: 1.8 g; Protein: 10.6 g; Cholesterol: 0 mg; Sodium: 308 mg

21.   Breakfast Buckwheat Muffins

Yield: 6 Servings
Total Time: 45 Minutes
Prep Time: 15 Minutes
Cook Time: 30 Minutes

Ingredients

- 1 cup buckwheat flour
- 1 teaspoon ground cinnamon
- 2 teaspoon baking powder
- 1/4 teaspoon coarse salt
- 4 free-range eggs
- 2 tablespoons raw honey
- 1 apple, peeled and diced

Directions

Preheat your oven to 350°F.

Line a standard muffin pan with paper liners and set aside.

Whisk together buckwheat flour, cinnamon, baking powder, and salt in a large bowl.

In a separate bowl, whisk together the eggs, and honey; pour the wet ingredients into the dry ingredients and fold in apple.

Scoop batter into the lined muffin cups and bake for about 30 minutes or until a tester comes out clean. Let the muffins cool on the wire rack before serving.

Nutritional Information Per Serving

Calories: 131; Total Fat: 3.6 g; Carbs: 20.6 g; Dietary fiber: 3.1 g; Sugars: 4.6 g; Protein: 6.3 g; Cholesterol: 109 mg; Sodium: 72 mg

22. Amaranth & Buckwheat Porridge

Yield: 4 Servings
Total Time: 20 Minutes
Prep Time: 10 minutes
Cook Time: 10 Minutes

Ingredients

- 1/3 cup amaranth
- 1/3 cup buckwheat groats
- 1 tablespoon fresh lemon juice
- 1 packet stevia
- 4 cups blackberries
- 1/2 teaspoon pure vanilla extract
- 1/4 teaspoon cinnamon
- 1/2 teaspoon ground cardamom
- Pinch of sea salt
- 2 cups water

Directions:

Mix amaranth and buckwheat in a bowl; cover with water and stir in a tablespoon of fresh lemon juice. Let soak for at least 8 hours or overnight. Drain and rinse well.

Blend together stevia and blackberries in a food processor until smooth; remove half of the puree to a plate and set aside.

Add buckwheat mixture, spices and ½ cup of water and puree until very smooth.

Transfer porridge to a saucepan and cook until thick. Serve into serving bowls and swirl in spoonfuls of blackberry puree; serve topped with more blackberries.

Nutritional Information Per Serving:

Calories: 160; Total Fat: 2.1 g; Carbs: 32.1 g; Dietary Fiber: 10.3 g; Sugars: 7.7 g; Protein: 5.7 g; Cholesterol: 0 mg; Sodium: 69 mg

23. Fish Breakfast Frittata

Yield: 2 Servings
Total Time: 30 Minutes
Prep Time: 10 Minutes
Cook Time: 20 Minutes

Ingredients:
- o 2 white fish fillets, diced
- o 1 tablespoon olive oil
- o 1 red onion, chopped
- o 1 green bell pepper, chopped
- o 2 garlic cloves, minced
- o ½ teaspoon turmeric powder
- o ½ teaspoon ground ginger
- o 1 teaspoon cumin
- o 6 free-range eggs beaten
- o Pinch of sea salt
- o 2 tablespoons chopped cilantro

Directions:

Preheat oven to 350°F.

Heat olive oil in oven-safe skillet and sauté red onion and green pepper; stir in garlic and cook for about 2 minutes or until fragrant.

Stir in cumin, turmeric, ginger, and salt; cook for about 1 minute.

Add in the fish and cover with eggs; season with salt and pepper and bake for about 15 minutes or until eggs are set.

Serve warm garnished with cilantro.

Nutritional Information per Serving:

Calories: 281; Total Fat: 16.2 g; Carbs: 5.8 g; Dietary Fiber: 1.5 g; Sugars: 2.5 g; Protein: 28 g; Cholesterol: 305 mg; Sodium: 205 mg

24.   Blueberry Buckwheat Pancakes

Yield: 6 Servings
Total Time: 26 Minutes
Prep Time: 10 Minutes
Cook Time: 16 Minutes

Ingredients

- 4 tablespoons olive oil
- 1 cup unsweetened almond milk
- 1 cup ground buckwheat flour
- ¼ teaspoon turmeric powder
- 1/8 teaspoon sea salt
- ½ inch ginger, grated
- 1 handful cilantro, chopped
- 1 red onion, chopped
- 1 cup fresh blueberries to serve

Directions

In a bowl, combine unsweetened almond milk, buckwheat, ginger, cilantro, and red onion until well combined.

Heat olive oil in a saucepan over medium low heat; add about ¼ cup of batter and spread out on the pan.

Cook for about 4 minutes per side or until golden brown. Transfer to a plate and keep warm; repeat with the remaining batter and oil.

Top the pancakes with fresh blueberries and fold into wraps. Serve with a glass of freshly squeezed lemon juice.

Nutritional Information per Serving:

Calories: 180; Total Fat: 11.1 g; Carbs: 18.4 g; Dietary Fiber: 5.1 g; Sugars: 2.9 g; Protein: 3.9 g; Cholesterol: 0 mg; Sodium: 72 mg

25.   Green Breakfast Smoothie

Yield: 3 Servings
Total Time: 5 Minutes
Prep Time: 5 Minutes
Cook Time: N/A

Ingredients

- 1 cup frozen cranberries
- 1 cup blackberries
- 1 cup chopped kale
- 1 cup chopped celery
- 1 cucumber
- 1 apple, diced
- 1 cup unsweetened almond milk
- 1/2 teaspoon ground turmeric
- 1/2 teaspoon ground cinnamon

Directions

In a blender, blend together apple, celery, cucumber, cranberries, blackberries, and rice milk until very smooth. Serve in a tall glass garnished with ground turmeric and cinnamon. Enjoy!

Nutritional Information per Serving:

Calories: 106; Total Fat: 1.6 g; Carbs: 21.8 g; Dietary Fiber: 6.6 g; Sugars: 11.4 g; Protein: 1.9 g; Cholesterol: 0 mg; Sodium: 71 mg

26.   Citrus & Pineapple Breakfast Shake

Yield: 4 Servings
Total Time: 5 Minutes
Prep Time: 5 Minutes
Cook Time: 0 Minutes

Ingredients
- 1 cup diced fresh pineapple
- 1 cup diced fresh mango
- ½ cup fresh grapefruit juice
- ½ cup lemon juice
- 1 teaspoon turmeric powder
- 1 cup unsweetened almond milk
- 1 cup frozen strawberries
- 1 cup blackberries
- 1 cup ice cubes

Directions
Combine all ingredients in a blender. Blend until very smooth.
Enjoy!

Nutritional Information per Serving:
Calories: 397; Total Fat: 2.7 g; Carbs: 26 g; Dietary Fiber: 11.1 g; Sugars: 13.4 g; Protein: 2.7 g; Cholesterol: 0 mg; Sodium: 105 mg

27.   Healthy Apple Green Smoothie

Yield: 2 Servings
Total Time: 5 Minutes
Prep Time: 5 Minutes
Cook Time: N/A

Ingredients

- 1 apple
- 1 cup fresh chopped kale
- 1 cucumber
- 1 cup unsweetened almond milk
- 1 tablespoon chopped mint
- 1 scoop protein powder
- 3/4 cup ice
- 1 tablespoon raw honey

Directions

Blend all the ingredients until smooth and thick.
Serve immediately!

Nutritional Information per Serving:

Calories: 176; Total Fat: 2.2 g; Carbs: 28.3 g; Dietary Fiber: 4.6 g; Sugars: 19.1 g;
Protein: 13.3 g; Cholesterol: 32 mg; Sodium: 91 mg

HEALTHY GALLBLADDER SURGERY DIET LUNCH RECIPES

28.   Avocado & Cucumber Salad with Toasted Nuts and Seeds

Yield: 4 Servings
Total Time: 15 Minutes
Prep Time: 15 Minutes
Cook Time: N/A

Ingredients

- 1 avocado, sliced
- 2 cucumbers, sliced
- 1 cup halved cherry tomatoes
- 3 cups chopped lettuce leaves
- 2 tablespoons fresh orange juice
- 1 tablespoon fresh grapefruit juice
- 1 clove garlic, minced
- A pinch of sea salt
- 1/2 cup extra virgin olive oil
- 1/2 cup toasted sunflower seeds
- 1/2 cup toasted cashews

Directions

Make Dressing: in a small bowl, whisk together orange juice, grapefruit juice, garlic, and salt; let sit for at least 10 minutes. Gradually whisk in extra virgin olive oil: set aside.

Add kale to another bowl and drizzle with a splash of the dressing; massage for about 2 minutes and let sit until tender.

Divide lettuce among serving plates and top each serving with cucumber, cherry tomatoes, and avocado.

Sprinkle with toasted cashews and sunflower seeds and drizzle generously with the dressing. Enjoy!

Nutritional Information per Serving:

Calories: 511; Total Fat: 46 g; Net Carbs: 19 g; Dietary Fiber: 6.2 g; Sugars: 8.2 g; Protein: 7 g; Cholesterol: 0 mg; Sodium: 87 mg

29.   Citrusy Soup with Caramelized Onions

Yield: 4 Servings
Total Time: 15 Minutes
Prep Time: 10 Minutes
Cook Time: 5 Minutes

Ingredients

- 3 tablespoons extra-virgin olive oil
- 1kg mushroom, trimmed
- 1 clove garlic, minced
- 4 red onions, chopped
- 4 cups vegetable stock
- 2 cups coconut milk
- 1 tablespoon fresh thyme
- 1/8 teaspoon sea salt
- Thyme sprigs
- 1/8 teaspoon pepper
- 2 lemons, juiced
- 2 oranges, juiced

Directions

Grill the mushrooms, turning frequently, for about 5 minutes or until charred and tender; set aside.

In a soup pot, sauté red onion in extra-virgin olive oil for about 8 minutes or until caramelized. Stir in vegetable stock and cook for a few minutes.

Place half of the caramelized onions and half of mushroom in a blender; blend until very smooth; add coconut milk, garlic, and thyme and continue blending until very smooth and creamy.

Return the soup to the pot and season with salt, thyme sprigs and pepper.

Remove from heat and stir in fresh lemon juice.

To serve, top with the remaining mushroom and caramelized onions!

Nutritional Information per Serving:

Calories: 325; Total Fat: 26.9 g; Net Carbs: 14 g; Dietary Fiber: 6.7 g; Sugars: 9.6 g; Protein: 8.6 g; Cholesterol: 0 mg; Sodium: 98 mg

30.   Lemon-Coconut Stir-Fried Greens

Yield: 2 Servings
Total Time: 20 Minutes
Prep Time: 10 Minutes
Cook Time: 10

Ingredients:

- o 2 tablespoons extra-virgin olive oil
- o 2 red onion, finely sliced
- o 2-3 garlic cloves, peeled and chopped
- o 1 piece of ginger, chopped
- o 2 cups squash, seeded, diced
- o 2 cups chopped spinach
- o 1 cup cabbage
- o 1 lemon, juiced
- o 1 tablespoon soy sauce
- o A pinch of sea salt
- o ½ cup coconut milk

Directions

In a large frying pan set over medium heat, heat olive oil; sauté onion for about 4 minutes or until fragrant.

Stir in garlic and ginger; cook for about 5 minutes, stirring.

Add squash and salt and cook until squash is tender.

Toss in the spinach, cabbage lemon juice, soy sauce, coconut milk, and sea salt; cook for 1 minute.

Nutritional Information Per Serving:

Calories: 376; Total Fat: 14.4 g; Net Carbs: 22.2 g; Dietary Fiber: 8.8 g; Sugars: 14.21 g; Protein: 7.2 g; Cholesterol: 0 mg; Sodium: 628 mg

31.   Crunchy Rainbow Detox Salad

Yield: 4 Servings
Total Time: 10 Minutes
Prep Time: 10 Minutes
Cook Time: N/A

Ingredients
For Lime Ginger Dressing
- ½ teaspoon ginger powder
- 1 teaspoon raw honey
- 1 tablespoon rice vinegar
- 2 tablespoons fresh lime juice

For Salad
- 1 cup carrot , shredded
- 1 cups shredded purple
- 1 cup shredded green cabbage
- 1 cup sliced beets
- 1 cup roughly chopped fresh parsley
- 2 tablespoons raisins
- 1 large avocado , sliced
- Toasted nuts for serving

Directions
Whisk together the dressing ingredients until well blended.

In a large bowl, toss together carrots, cabbage, and parsley; top with raisins, toasted nuts, and sliced avocado and drizzle with the dressing.

Let marinate for at least 5 minutes before serving.

Nutritional Information per Serving:
Calories: 154 Total Fat: 9.9 g; Carbs: 16.7 g; Dietary Fiber: 5.8 g; Sugars: 7.4 g; Protein: 2.2 g; Cholesterol: 0 mg; Sodium: 37 mg

32. Delicious Green Soup with Brown Rice

Yield: 4 Servings
Total Time: 1 Hour 15 Minutes
Prep Time: 15 Minutes
Cook Time: 60 Minutes

Ingredients

- 2 cups chopped kale
- 3 cups baby spinach
- 1 cup brown rice, rinsed
- 2 yellow onions, chopped
- 2 tablespoons olive oil
- 3 cups water
- 4 cups homemade vegetable broth
- 1/2 cup fresh lemon juice
- 1/4 teaspoon sea salt

Directions

Add the two tablespoons of olive oil in a large pan and cook the onions over medium heat. Sprinkle with salt and cook for 5 minutes until they start browning.

Lower the heat and pour in two tablespoons of water. Cover and lover the heat and cook for 25 minutes until the onions caramelize, stirring frequently.

Meanwhile, add the remaining water and some salt to a Dutch oven and stir in the rice. Bring to a boil then lower the heat and simmer for about 15 minutes until tender. Stir in the kale into the cooked rice, cover and cook for 10 more minutes.

Add the onions to the rice mixture together with the broth and spinach and simmer for 5 minutes.

Use an immersion blender to puree the rice mixture until smooth then stir in the lemon juice.

Serve into soup bowls and drizzle each with some olive oil.

Nutritional Information per Serving:

Calories: 323; Total Fat: 6.7 g; Net Carbs: 33.5 g; Dietary Fiber: 10.1 g; Sugars: 4.1 g; Protein: 10.1 g; Cholesterol: 0 mg; Sodium: 619 mg

33.   Avocado &Mixed Veggie Salad with Garlic Vinaigrette

Yield: 2 Servings
Total Time: 15 Minutes
Prep Time: 15 Minutes
Cook Time: N/A

Ingredients

- 4 cups chopped kale
- 1 cup snow peas, chopped
- 1 red bell pepper, chopped
- 1 carrot, peeled and cut into ribbons using a julienne peeler
- 1 cup edamame
- 1 shallot, finely sliced
- A handful each of basil and cilantro, chopped
- 1 avocado, cubed
- 1/4 teaspoon sea salt

For the vinaigrette:

- ¼ cup extra-virgin olive oil
- 1 tablespoon very finely grated fresh ginger
- 2 teaspoons freshly squeezed lime juice
- 3 cloves garlic minced
- 2 tablespoons apple cider vinegar

Directions

Place the kale in a large bowl and sprinkle with the sea salt. Gently massage the kale using your hands until soft and fragrant.

Toss in the remaining salad ingredients until well combined.

Whisk the vinaigrette ingredients then drizzle over the salad and toss well to combine.

Nutritional Information per Serving:

Calories: 389; Total Fat: 27 g; Net Carbs: 20.3 g; Dietary Fiber: 9.2 g; Sugars: 4.6 g; Protein: 13.5g; Cholesterol: 0 mg; Sodium: 174

34.   Stir-Fried Tofu and Veggies

Yield: 4 Servings
Total Time: 25 Minutes
Prep Time: 15 Minutes
Cook Time: 10 Minutes

Ingredients for

- 250g green beans
- 3 medium zucchinis
- 1 pound firm tofu
- 1 green bell pepper
- 1 red bell pepper
- 3 tomatoes

- 2 tablespoons coconut oil
- 2 cups coconut milk
- ¼ tablespoon ginger
- ½ tablespoon curry powder
- A pinch of sea salt

Directions

Dice zucchinis, tofu, bell peppers, tomatoes and beans in bite-size pieces. Heat oil in a pan and fry tofu for about 3 minutes. Add beans, zucchini, and bell peppers; fry for 3 minutes more.

Stir in coconut milk and tomatoes and cook for a few minutes. Season with ginger, curry powder, and salt. Serve with steamed brown rice.

Nutritional Information Per Serving:

Calories: 493; Total Fat: 40.9 g; Net Carbs: 16.2 g; Dietary Fiber: 9.7 g; Sugars: 12.8 g; Protein: 16.5 g; Cholesterol: 0 mg; Sodium: 115 mg

35. Super Healthy Salad with Lemony Dressing

Yield: 6 Servings
Total Time: 10 Minutes
Prep Time: 10 Minutes
Cook Time: N/A

Ingredients

For Lemony Dressing

- ½ cup fresh lemon juice
- 6 tablespoons water
- ½-inch knob of ginger, minced
- 1 tablespoon Dijon mustard
- 1½ tablespoons raw honey
- 1 clove garlic, chopped
- ¼ teaspoon salt
- 1 tablespoon poppy seeds

For the Salad

- 1 cup carrots, roughly chopped
- 2 cups red cabbage, roughly chopped
- 2 cups Brussels sprouts, roughly chopped
- 2 cups broccoli florets
- 2 cups kale
- 2 tablespoons toasted sunflower seeds
- ½ cup toasted almonds, chopped
- ½ cup chopped parsley

Directions

In a blender, blend together all the ingredients, except poppy seeds until smooth; add poppy seeds and set aside.

Mix all the salad ingredients in a large bowl; drizzle with the dressing and toss to coat well. Serve.

Nutrition Information per Serving

Calories: 175; Total Fat: 11.8 g; Carbs: 15.4 g; Dietary Fiber; 4.7 g; Sugars: 5.6 g; Protein: 5.3 g Cholesterol: 0 mg; Sodium: 27 mg

36.   Healthy Superfood Salad with Lemon-Tahini Dressing

Yield: 2 Servings
Total Time: 10 Minutes
Prep Time: 10 Minutes

Ingredients
For the Salad

- 1 large cucumber, chopped
- ½ cup shredded carrot
- 2 green onions, sliced
- 1 cup Romaine lettuce, chopped
- 1 cup baby spinach, chopped
- ½ cup snap peas, sliced
- ½ cup blueberries
- ½ cup avocado, sliced
- 1 tablespoon chia seeds

For the Dressing

- 1 tablespoon tahini
- 1 teaspoon sesame oil
- 1 tablespoon lemon juice
- 1 tablespoon rice wine vinegar
- 1 teaspoon raw honey
- ¼ teaspoon oregano
- 1 clove garlic, minced
- ¼ teaspoon sea salt

Directions

Combine all the salad ingredients in a large bowl.

Whisk together all the dressing ingredients in a small bowl until well blended.

Drizzle the dressing over the salad and toss until well coated.

Enjoy!

Nutritional Information per Serving:

Calories: 256; Total Fat: 14.1 g; Carbs: 29.7 g; Dietary Fiber: 8.5 g; Sugars: 13.5 g; Protein: 6.5 g; Cholesterol: 0 mg; Sodium: 343 mg

37.   Crunchy Superfood Cleanse Salad

Yields: 4 Servings
Total Time: 10 Minutes
Prep Time: 10 Minutes
Cook Time: N/A

Ingredients
- 1 cup fresh blueberries
- 1 cup shredded carrots
- 5 cups baby spinach
- 12 toasted almonds, sliced
- 2 dates, pitted and diced
- 1 tablespoon fresh lemon juice
- 2 tablespoons extra-virgin olive oil

Directions
Mix all the ingredients, except lemon juice and olive oil, in a large bowl.

Whisk together olive oil and lemon juice and pour over the salad; toss to combine well and serve.

Nutritional Information per Serving:
Calories: 180; Total Fat: 9 g; Carbs: 25 g; Dietary Fiber: 4 g; Sugars: 18 g; Protein: 3 g; Cholesterol: 0 mg; Sodium: 46 mg

38.   Crunchy Vegetable Sauté

Yield: 2 Servings
Total Time: 19 Minutes
Prep Time: 5 Minutes
Cook Time: 14 Minutes

Ingredients

- o 2 tablespoons extra-virgin olive oil
- o 2 cups green beans, sliced
- o 1 cup chopped red onion
- o 2 garlic cloves
- o 2 medium zucchini, thinly sliced
- o A pinch of salt
- o 2 tablespoons lemon juice
- o 2 tablespoons sliced scallions
- o 1 cup sliced toasted almonds

Method

Add olive oil to a skillet set over medium heat.

Stir in red onions for about 5 minutes or until fragrant; add in garlic, green beans, zucchini, sea salt and pepper and sauté, stirring, for about 9 minutes or until the veggies are crisp tender.

Remove the pan from heat and stir in lemon juice and scallions.

Serve topped with sliced toasted almonds.

Nutritional Information per Serving:

Calories: 493; Total Fat: 38.4 g; Net Carbs: 18.3 g; Dietary Fiber: 13.4 g; Sugars: 9.9 g; Protein: 15.5 g; Cholesterol: 0 mg; Sodium: 111 mg

39. Black Bean Soup

Yield: 6 Servings
Total Time: 1 Hour 10 Minutes
Prep Time: 10 Minutes
Cook Time: 1 Hour

Ingredients

- 6 cups boiling water
- 1 large red onion, diced
- 1 pound dried black beans
- 1 teaspoon sea salt
- 1 cup salsa
- 12 ounces frozen corn kernels
- 1 tablespoon fresh lime juice
- Avocado slices
- baked Whole-wheat tortilla chips

Directions

Boil water in an instant pot and turn it to sauté setting; add onion and cook, stirring often, until tender and browned.

Stir in beans, boiling water, and sea salt; turn off the sauté function. Lock lid in place and turn on high pressure, adjusting time to 30 minutes. Let pressure come down naturally before opening the pot.

Remove about 3 cups of beans to a blender and blend until very smooth; return to pot and add salsa and corn.

Adjust seasoning and turn the pot on sauté; cook until heated through. Ladle in serving bowls and drizzle with lime juice, garnish with avocado slices and serve with baked tortilla chips.

Nutritional Information per Serving:

Calories: 329; Total Fat: 1 g; Carbs: 65 g; Dietary Fiber: 15 g; Sugars: 7 g; Protein: 18 g; Cholesterol: 0 mg; Sodium: 707 mg

40.   Healthy Vegetable Salad

Yield: 4 Servings
Total Time: 10 Minutes
Prep Time: 10 Minutes
Cook Time: N/A

For salad:
- 1/2 small head red cabbage, shredded
- 1/2 small head Napa cabbage, shredded
- 1/4 cup arugula
- 4 cups fresh baby spinach
- 5 large radish, shredded
- 2 large carrots, shredded
- 1/4 cup pistachios
- 1/4 cup chopped parsley
- 1 cup fresh basil leaves
- 1 teaspoon lemon zest

For dressing:
- 3 tablespoons extra virgin olive oil
- 1/3 cup shallots
- 2/3 cup apple cider vinegar
- 1 teaspoon chia seeds
- 1/4 cup pure raw honey
- 2 tablespoons freshly squeezed lemon juice

Directions

In a large bowl, combine all salad ingredients and set aside.

In a skillet, whisk together dressing ingredients and cook for about 15 minutes; remove from heat and pour over the salad. Toss and serve right away.

Nutritional Information per Serving:

Calories: 292; Total Fat: 15.2 g; Carbs: 35.5 g; Dietary Fiber: 9.5 g; Sugars: 20.2 g; Protein: 6.6 g; Cholesterol: 0 mg; Sodium: 115 mg

41.   Cleansing Superfood Salad

Yield: 6 Servings
Total Time: 10 Minutes
Prep Time: 10 Minutes
Cook Time: N/A

Ingredients
For the dressing:
- 2 teaspoons whole-grain mustard
- 1 tablespoon freshly grated ginger
- 1/2 cup fresh lemon juice
- 1 teaspoonolive oil
- 1 teaspoon raw honey
- 1/4 teaspoon salt

For the salad:
- 2 cups broccoli florets
- 2 cups red cabbage, thinly sliced
- 2 cups chopped kale
- 1 cup grated carrot
- 1 red bell pepper, sliced into strips
- 2 avocados, diced
- 1/2 cup chopped parsley
- 1 cup walnuts
- 1 tablespoon sesame seeds

Directions
In a blender, blend all the dressing ingredients until well blended; set aside.
In a salad bowl, mix broccoli, cabbage, kale, carrots and bell pepper; pour the dressing over the salad and toss until well coated.
Add diced avocado, parsley, walnuts and sesame seed; toss again to coat and serve.

Nutritional Information per Serving:
Calories: 437; Total Fat: 38.7 g; Carbs: 19.6 g; Dietary Fiber: 8.9 g; Sugars: 5.2 g; Protein: 9.1 g; Cholesterol: 0 mg; Sodium: 153 mg

42.   Avocado, Cucumber &Tomato Salad

Yield: 4 Servings
Total Time: 10 Minutes
Prep Time: 10 Minutes
Cook Time: N/A

Ingredients

- 1 large avocado, sliced
- 2 cucumbers, sliced
- 1 red onion, thinly sliced
- 1 large fennel bulb, chopped
- 4 medium tomatoes, chopped
- 1 tablespoon avocado oil
- 3 tablespoons extra virgin olive oil
- 2 tablespoons fresh lime juice
- 2 tablespoons chopped fresh cilantro
- 1/8 teaspoon sea salt

Directions

In a bowl, combine avocado, red onion, fennel, and tomatoes.
In a small bowl, whisk together avocado oil, extra virgin olive oil, lime juice, cilantro, and salt; pour over the avocado mixture and toss to combine well. Enjoy!

Nutritional Information Per Serving:

Calories: 231; Total Fat: 21 g; Net Carbs: 6.3 g; Dietary Fiber: 5.7 g; Sugars: 4.7 g; Protein: 2.4 g; Cholesterol: 0 mg; Sodium: 70 mg

43. Mushroom &Buckwheat Dish

Yield: 6 Servings
Total Time: 55 Minutes
Prep Time: 20 Minutes
Cook Time: 35 Minutes

Ingredients

- 1 cup uncooked buckwheat
- 2 cup water
- 2 cups mushrooms
- 1 red onion, chopped
- 1 cup chopped green onions
- 3 tablespoons coconut oil
- A pinch of salt

Directions

Combine buckwheat, salt, and water in a pan   bring to a boil; cook for 25 minutes or until liquid is absorbed.

Melt coconut oil in a pan and fry in red onion until tender; stir in mushrooms and cook for about 5 minutes or until golden brown.

Stir in cooked buckwheat and remove from heat. Serve topped with freshly chopped green onions.

Nutrition info Per Serving:

Calories: 166; Total Fat: 6.8 g; Net Carbs: 20.1 g; Dietary Fiber: 3.9 g; Sugars: 1.6; Protein: 5.1 g; Cholesterol: 15 mg; Sodium: 48 mg

44. Lunch Millet Lettuce Wraps

Yield: 2 Servings
Total Time: 30 Minutes
Prep Time: 10 Minutes
Cook Time: 20 Minutes

Ingredients

- 4 leaves lettuce
- ¼ cup millet
- 1 teaspoon coconut oil
- ½ cup water
- ¼ red onion, chopped
- 1 clove garlic, minced
- 2 tablespoons fresh lime juice
- 1 teaspoon chopped cilantro
- ½ teaspoon sea salt
- 1 carrot, chopped

Directions

In a skillet, toast millet for about 5 minutes or until fragrant and toasted; transfer to a plate and set aside. Add coconut oil to the skillet and sauté in red onion and garlic for about 3 minutes or until fragrant. Stir in toasted millet, lime juice, cilantro, sea salt and water; simmer for about 10 minutes or until the liquid is absorbed. Remove from heat. Divide carrots among the lettuce leaves and top each with the millet mixture. Roll to form wraps and serve.

Nutrition info Per Serving:

Calories: 133; Total Fat: 3 g; Net Carbs: 19.9 g; Dietary Fiber: 3.3 g; Sugars: 2.2; Protein: 3.3 g; Cholesterol: 5 mg; Sodium: 507 mg

45.   Millet Stir Fry with Veggies

Yield: 2 Servings
Total Time: 30 Minutes
Prep Time: 20 Minutes
Cook Time: 20 Minutes

Ingredients

- 1 cup millet
- 1 red onion, chopped
- 1 tablespoon grated ginger
- 2 cloves garlic, minced
- 1/2 cup chopped red and green bell peppers
- 1/2 cup chopped French beans
- 1/2 cup chopped carrots
- 1 teaspoon coriander powder
- 1 teaspoon cumin powder
- 1 teaspoon turmeric powder
- Salt to taste
- 1 tablespoon olive oil
- fresh coriander leaves

Directions

Wash millet under running water and soak for at least 10 minutes.

Meanwhile, heat oil in a pot and cook in garlic and gingerfor 1 minute; stir in onions and spices and cook for 2 minutes.

Rinse the millet and drain; add to the pot along with two cups of water. Cover and cook for about 10 minutes or until liquid is absorbed and millet is tender. Fluff and serve topped with fresh coriander.

Nutritional Information per Serving:

Calories: 327; Total Fat: 6.4 g; Net Carbs: 35.8 g; Dietary Fiber: 11.7 g; Sugars: 2 g
Protein: 10.7g; Cholesterol: 0 mg; Sodium: 58 mg

46. Veggie Salad with Toasted Pumpkin Seeds

Yield: 2 Servings
Total Time: 5 Minutes
Prep Time: 5 Minutes
Cook Time: N/A

Ingredients:
- 4 ounces spinach
- 2 watermelon radishes, thinly sliced
- 1 small yellow squash, thinly sliced
- 1 small yellow or red beet, thinly sliced
- 1 small cucumber, thinly sliced
- 1 small carrot, thinly sliced
- 1 tablespoon toasted pumpkin seeds
- 1 tablespoon extra-virgin olive oil
- 1 lemon, juiced
- sea salt, to taste
- ground pepper, to taste

Directions:
Combine veggies in a large bowl and toss with lemon juice and olive oil; season with salt and pepper and serve right away.

Nutritional Information per Serving:
Calories: 159; Total Fat: 9.6 g; Carbs: 17.3 g; Dietary Fiber: 4.4 g; Sugars: 8.6 g; Protein: 5.4 g; Cholesterol: 0 mg; Sodium: 225 mg

47.   Sweet Potato & Scallion Salad

Yield: 4 Servings
Total Time: 20 Minutes
Prep Time: 10 Minutes
Cook Time: 10 Minutes

Ingredients

- 4 large sweet potatoes, peeled, diced
- 1 cup sliced scallions
- 1 medium red bell pepper, chopped
- 2 tablespoons minced mint leaves
- 1 tablespoon grated orange zest
- 2 teaspoons ground cumin
- ¼ cup apple cider vinegar
- 4 tablespoons extra-virgin olive oil
- ¼ teaspoon sea salt

Directions

Preheat your oven to 350 degrees.

Place sweet potatoes on a baking sheet and drizzle with half of oil; sprinkle with salt and pepper and toss to coat well. Bake in the preheated oven for about 30 minutes or until tender and browned.

Meanwhile, add the remaining oil to the blender along with bell pepper, vinegar, zest, and cumin, sea salt, pepper and blend until very smooth.

Remove the potatoes from the oven and toss with mint and scallions.

Drizzle with the dressing and toss to coat well. Enjoy!

Nutrition info Per Serving:

Calories: 325; Total Fat: 14.6 g; Net Carbs: 39.5 g; Dietary Fiber: 7.7 g; Sugars: 2.9; Protein: 3.4 g; Cholesterol: 0 mg; Sodium: 139 mg

48.   Super Cleansing Lunch Salad

Yield: 5 Servings
Total Time: 25 Minutes
Prep Time: 10 Minutes
Cook Time: 15 Minutes

Ingredients:

- 2 heads broccoli
- 1 head cauliflower
- 2 ½ cups shredded carrots
- 1/2 cup raisins
- 1 cup currants
- 1/2 cup sunflower seeds
- 1/2 cup chopped parsley
- ¾ cup fresh lemon juice
- ½ teaspoon kosher salt
- 1 tablespoon raw honey

Directions

Chop broccoli in a food processor until fine; transfer to a large bowl.
Chop cauliflower in a food processor until fine; add to the bowl with broccoli.
Stir in shredded carrots, raisins, currants, sunflower seeds, and parsley.
Add fresh lemon juice and season. Drizzle with honey add toss to coat well. Serve immediately.

Nutritional Information per Serving:

Calories: 153 Total Fat: 3 g; Carbs: 30.1 g; Dietary Fiber: 5.9 g; Sugars: 18.1 g; Protein: 4.7 g; Cholesterol: 0 mg; Sodium: 312 mg

49. Healthy Lentil Soup

Yield: 6 Servings
Total Time: 45 Minutes
Prep Time: 10 Minutes
Cook Time: 35 Minutes

Ingredients

- 6 cups homemade vegetable broth
- 2 tablespoons minced garlic
- 1 1/2 cups chopped red onion
- 1 teaspoon paprika
- 1 teaspoon ground coriander
- ½ teaspoon ground pepper
- 1 1/2 cups red lentils
- 1 1/2-2 cups chopped carrots
- Fresh lemon juice
- Fresh cilantro, chopped

Directions

Add vegetable stock to a saucepan and stir in garlic, onion, paprika, coriander and ground pepper; bring to a gentle boil. Boil for about 5 minutes and then add in lentils; simmer for about 15 minutes and then add in chopped carrots. Cook, covered, for 15 minutes more or until lentils are tender. Serve in bowls garnished with fresh lemon and chopped cilantro. Enjoy!

Nutrition Information per Serving

Calories: 213; Total Fat: 0.6 g; Carbs: 36.5 g; Dietary Fiber: 16.2 g; Sugars: 3.6 g; Protein: 15.2 g Cholesterol: 0 mg; Sodium: 94 mg

50.   Sweet Beet Salad with Toasted Pumpkin Seeds

Yield: 4 Servings
Total Time: 25 Minutes
Prep Time: 10 Minutes
Cook Time: 15 Minutes

Ingredients

- 1½ pounds red beets, peeled and sliced into ½-inch pieces
- 1 ½ cups sliced red onion
- 2 large tangerines, sectioned
- 6 cups loosely packed baby arugula
- 2 tablespoons balsamic vinegar
- ¼ cup toasted pumpkin seeds

Directions

Add the beets to a saucepan and cover with water; bring to a gentle boil and then simmer for about 15 minutes or until tender.

Meantime, add red onion to another saucepan and cook over medium high heat for about 5 minutes or until lightly browned, adding water to prevent sticking; transfer to a bowl.

Drain the beets and let cool; add to a bowl with onions and add in tangerines, arugula, and balsamic vinegar; toss to coat and sprinkle with toasted pumpkin seeds. Enjoy!

Nutritional Information per Serving:

Calories: 394; Total Fat: 5.4 g; Carbs: 80.8 g; Dietary Fiber: 15.1 g; Sugars: 63.3 g; Protein: 18.8 g; Cholesterol: 0 mg; Sodium: 498 mg

51.   Lunch Turkey Lettuce Wraps

Yield: 4 Servings
Total Time: 25 Minutes
Prep Time: 15 Minutes
Cook Time: 10 Minutes

Ingredients

- 500g ground turkey
- 2 teaspoons extra-virgin olive oil
- 2 cups shredded cabbage
- 1 large carrot, grated
- 1/2 cup chopped green beans
- 2 garlic cloves, chopped
- 1/2 red onion, chopped
- 2 spring onions, sliced
- 2 tablespoons chopped coriander
- 1 iceberg lettuce, halved, cored

Directions

Heat a skillet over medium high heat; cook in ground turkey, stirring to break up the turkey with a spoon for about 5 minutes or until cooked through. Transfer to a dish. Add oil to the pan and sauté red onions and garlic until fragrant and then stir in green beans for about 3 minutes.

Return the turkey and cook for about 1 minute or until flavors blend; stir in carrots, cabbage, spring onions, and pepper and then remove the pan from the heat.

Divide the lettuce leaves among four serving plates and spoon the turkey mixture onto each serving. Top each with coriander and the remaining spring onions. Enjoy!

Nutritional Information per Serving:

Calories: 283; Total Fat: 10.2 g; Carbs: 7.2 g; Dietary Fiber: 2.3 g; Sugars: 3 g; Protein: 39.2 g; Cholesterol: 112 mg; Sodium: 104 mg

52. Chicken & Zucchini Soup

Yield: 4 Servings
Total Time: 20 Minutes
Prep Time: 10 Minutes
Cook Time: 10 Minutes

Ingredients

- 450g skinless chicken breast fillets, halved
- 1 tablespoon olive oil
- 2 garlic cloves, crushed
- 3 cups zucchini noodles
- 1/2 cup coconut cream
- 1/3 cup homemade chicken broth
- 1 tablespoon fresh dill leaves
- 2 tablespoons fresh chives, chopped
- 1 cup kale

Directions

Coat a pan with oil and set over medium high heat; season chicken with salt and pepper and cook in the pan for about 3 minutes per side or until cooked through; transfer to a plate and keep warm.

Add oil to the pan and sauté garlic until fragrant; stir in zucchini noodles and cook for about 2 minutes; stir in coconut cream and chicken broth and simmer for about 2 minutes or until tender.

Slice the chicken and add to the zucchini sauce along with chives and dill. Divide among serving bowls and top each with kale.

Enjoy!

Nutritional Information per Serving:

Calories: 207; Total Fat: 8.3 g; Carbs: 6.6 g; Dietary Fiber: 1.4 g; Sugars: 2.2 g; Protein: 26.3 g; Cholesterol: 78 mg; Sodium: 148 mg

53. Crunchy Steak Salad

Yield: 2 Servings
Total Time: 15 Minutes
Prep Time: 10 Minutes
Cook Time: 5 Minutes

Ingredients

- 250g steak
- 1 tablespoon tamari soy sauce
- 1 tablespoon olive oil
- 1 tablespoon olive oil
- 1/2 tablespoon lemon juice
- 4 radishes, sliced
- 1/2 red bell pepper, sliced
- 2 cups salad greens
- 1/2 cup toasted cashews

Directions

Pour tamari sauce in a large bowl; add in steak and toss to coat well; cover and let marinate for a few hours before cooking.

In another bowl, combine green salad, radishes, bell peppers, lemon juice, and olive oil; toss to coat well and set aside.

Heat olive oil in a skillet over medium-high heat; cook the steak for about 8 minutes per side or until cooked through and browned on the outside. Remove from heat and let cool for a minute before slicing to serve. Divide the salad between two plates and top each with steak slices and toasted cashews.

Nutritional Information per Serving:

Calories: 421; Total Fat: 20.4 g; Carbs: 10.1 g; Dietary Fiber: 3.6 g; Sugars: 1.9 g; Protein: 49.5 g; Cholesterol: 113 mg; Sodium: 604 mg

54.   Delicious Turkey Soup

Yield: 2 Servings
Total Time: 40 Minutes
Prep Time: 10 Minutes
Cook Time: 30 Minutes

Ingredients

- 1 teaspoons extra-virgin olive oil
- 1 red onion, finely sliced
- 1 ginger, finely chopped
- 1 clove garlic, finely chopped
- 1 lemon grass, bashed with a rolling pin
- ½ cup chopped green beans
- 1 cup water
- ½ cup vegetable stock
- 8 oz. turkey, cooked, roughly chopped
- 1/8 teaspoon sea salt
- 1 cup coriander, finely chopped
- 1 cup kale, roughly chopped
- 2 tablespoons fresh lime juice

Directions

Add olive oil to a medium pan set over medium heat; stir in red onions and sauté for about 5 minutes or until translucent. Add ginger and garlic and sauté for about 3 minutes or until garlic is golden.

Stir in lemon grass, green beans, milk, and vegetable sock; bring to a simmer. Simmer for about 15 minutes or until green beans is soft.

Stir in turkey and salt; cook for about 5 minutes or until turkey is cooked heated through. Remove from heat and stir in coriander and kale; serve into soup bowls and sprinkle with a squeeze of lime juice and coriander.

Nutritional Information per Serving:

Calories: 346; Total Fat: 15.4 g; Carbs: 16.5 g; Dietary Fiber: 3.9 g; Sugars: 4.4 g; Protein: 36.6 g; Cholesterol: 86 mg; Sodium: 237 mg

55.   Stir-Fried Chicken& Veggies

Yield: 4 Servings
Total Time: 20 Minutes
Prep Time: 10 Minutes
Cook Time: 10 Minutes

Ingredients:

- 1 pound skinless chicken breasts, thinly sliced strips
- 4 cups diced cremini mushrooms
- 4 tablespoons fresh lemon juice
- Pinch of sea salt
- 3 teaspoons extra-virgin olive oil
- 1 large yellow onion, thinly chopped
- 1/2 red bell pepper, sliced
- 1/2 green bell pepper, sliced

Directions:

Place the chicken in a bowl; stir in lemon juice and sea salt. Toss to coat well.

Heat a tablespoon of olive oil in a pan set over medium high heat.

Add chicken and cook for about 1 minute or until meat is browned; stir for another 2 minutes and then remove from heat.

Heat the remaining oil to the pan and sauté onions for about 2 minutes or until caramelized; stir in mushrooms for about 5 minutes and then stir in peppers; cook for 2 minutes more and return chicken to pan.

 Serve hot!

Nutritional Information per Serving:

Calories: 322; Total Fat: 16 g; Carbs: 9.3 g; Dietary Fiber: 1.8 g; Sugars: 4.7 g; Protein: 33.7 g; Cholesterol: 81 mg; Sodium: 163 mg

56.   Superfood Avocado Salad with Citrus Dressing

Yield: 8 Servings
Total Time: 10 Minutes
Prep Time: 10 Minutes
Cook Time: N/A

Ingredients
For the dressing
- 1/2 cup olive oil
- 1 teaspoon raw honey
- 3 tablespoons fresh lemon juice
- 2 tablespoons lime juice
- 1 tablespoon apple cider vinegar
- ½ teaspoon finely grated lemon zest
- 1 teaspoon Dijon mustard
- 1 garlic clove, crushed
- 2 teaspoons freshly grated ginger

For the salad
- 1 cup watercress, large stalks removed and chopped
- 1 cup lamb's lettuce, chopped
- 1/2 cup chopped chicory
- 3 lemon, peeled, segmented, and deseeded
- 1 avocado

Directions
In a jar, combine all dressing ingredients and shake to mix well. Chill in the refrigerator for at least 2 days before using.

Combine all salad ingredients and chill for at least 1 hour.

When ready, drizzle with dressing and mix to coat well. Enjoy!

Nutritional Information per Serving:
Calories: 132; Total Fat: 13.7 g; Carbs: 3.4 g; Dietary Fiber: 0.8 g; Sugars: 0.9 g; Protein: 0.4 g; Cholesterol: 0 mg; Sodium: 10 mg

57.   Super Cleansing Salad

Yield: 3 Servings
Total Time: 10 Minutes
Prep Time: 10 Minutes
Cook Time: N/A

Ingredients

- 1 small red onion, sliced into thin rings
- 1 cup watercress, rinsed
- 1 zucchini, shaved
- 1 small broccoli head, rinsed and cut in small florets
- 1 avocado, diced
- ½ teaspoon Dijon mustard
- 2 tablespoon s fresh lemon juice
- 1 tablespoon extra-virgin olive oil
- ½ teaspoon sea salt
- ¼ cup crushed toasted almonds
- 1 tablespoon chia seeds

Directions

In a large bowl, mix together the veggies until well combined.

In a small bowl, whisk together lemon juice, olive oil, mustard and salt until well blended; pour over the salad and toss until well coated. Add almonds and chia seeds and toss to combine. Set the salad aside for at least 5 minutes for flavors to combine before serving.

Nutritional Information per Serving:

Calories: 228; Total Fat: 18.8 g; Carbs: 13.6 g; Dietary Fiber: 8.2 g; Sugars: 2.7 g; Protein: 5.1 g; Cholesterol: 0 mg; Sodium: 265 mg

58.   Delicious Mung& Veggie Stew with Avocado

Yield: 3 Servings
Total Time: 20 Minutes
Prep Time: 5 Minutes
Cook Time: 15 Minutes

Ingredients

- 2 teaspoon sesame oil
- ½ cup diced carrots
- ½ cup chopped celery
- 1 cup chopped leeks
- 2 garlic cloves, minced
- 1 teaspoon minced ginger
- 1 tablespoon date paste
- 2 tablespoons walnut paste
- 2 tablespoons fresh lime juice
- 1/4 teaspoon cardamom powder
- 1/2 teaspoon se salt
- 4 cups vegetable broth
- 1 cup chopped spinach
- 2 cups cooked mung beans
- 1 avocado, diced
- ½ cup chopped parsley

Directions

Heat oil in a stock pot over medium high heat.

Sauté chopped veggies and seasonings except spinach.

Cook for about 10 minutes and then stir in, vegetable broth, spinach and mung beans; simmer for about 3 minutes and remove from heat.

Serve the stew with small avocado cubes, garnished with tomatoes and parsley.

Nutritional Information per Serving:

Calories: 497; Total Fat: 19.7 g; Net Carbs: 29.8 g; Dietary Fiber: 18.6 g; Sugars: 9.9 g; Protein: 20.7 g; Cholesterol: 0 mg; Sodium: 505 mg

59.   Crunchy Fried Tofu with Greens

Yields: 4 Servings
Total Time: 35 Minutes
Prep Time: 10 Minutes
Cook Time: 25 Minutes

Ingredients

- 2 tablespoons extra virgin olive oil
- 400g extra-firm tofu, sliced
- 2 red onions, thinly sliced
- 2 medium red bell peppers, chopped
- 2 teaspoons grated fresh ginger
- 4 cup spring greens, chopped
- 4 tablespoons teriyaki sauce
- 1 cup toasted cashews, chopped

Directions

Add half oil to a pan set over medium heat. Add tofu and fry until golden. Transfer to a plate.

Add the remaining oil to the pan and sauté onion until translucent.

Stir in bell pepper and continue sautéing until onion is tender and golden. Stir in ginger and greens until wilted.

Stir in tofu and season with teriyaki sauce. Top with toasted cashews to serve.

Nutritional Information per Serving:

Calories: 416; Total Fat: 29 g; Net Carbs: 22.9 g; Dietary Fiber: 5 g; Sugars: 10.3 g; Protein: 18.3 g; Cholesterol: 0 mg; Sodium: 793 mg

60.   Scrumptious Ratatouille

Yield: 4 Servings
Total Time: 1 Hour 20 Minutes
Prep Time: 20 Minutes
Cook Time: 1 Hour

Ingredients

- 1/4 teaspoon apple cider vinegar
- 1 tablespoon extra-virgin olive oil
- 1 cup crushed tomatoes
- 1/4 teaspoon chili powder
- 1 teaspoon herbs de Provence
- 1 tablespoon chopped fresh basil
- 1 teaspoon minced garlic
- 1/4 teaspoon salt
- 4 large fresh tomatoes, sliced
- 2 large eggplants, sliced
- 2 large zucchinis, sliced
- 2 red onions, chopped

Directions

Preheat your oven to 350°F and lightly grease a 6 by 9-inch baking dish.

In a bowl, mix together vinegar, oil and crushed tomatoes until well combined; stir in chili powder, herbs de Provence, basil, garlic and salt and pour the mixture into the prepared baking dish. Spread it into a single layer and smoothen the top.

In alternative pattern, layer vegetable slices on top of the tomato mixture in rows repeating the layers until you have used all the veggies. Spray the veggies with oil and bake in the oven for about 1 hour or until the tomato sauce is bubbly and veggies tender. Serve hot garnished with chopped basil.

Nutritional Information per Serving:

Calories: 206; Total Fat: 4.7 g; Net Carbs: 12.3 g; Dietary Fiber: 16.9 g; Sugars: 21.7 g; Protein: 8.4 g; Cholesterol: 0 mg; Sodium: 302 mg;

61. Superfood Toasted Almonds Wraps

Yield: 3 Servings
Total Time: 20 Minutes
Prep Time: 20 Minutes
Cook Time: N/A

Ingredients

- 6 collard leaves
- 1 cup pecans, toasted
- 1 cup toasted almonds
- 1 ripe avocado, sliced
- 1/3 cup alfalfa sprouts
- 1 red pepper, sliced
- 1 lemon
- 1 tablespoon extra-virgin olive oil
- 1 teaspoon cumin
- 1 teaspoon grated ginger
- 1 tablespoon tamari

Directions

Cut off the stems from the collard leaves and rinse them under running water to remove any grit.

Soak them in warm water with the juice of half a lemon for about 10 minutes then dry the leaves using paper towels.

Shave of the central root so the leaves become easier to roll.

Add the toasted nuts, cumin, and tamari, ginger and olive oil to your food processor and pulse until the mixture forms a ball-like shape.

Spread out the collard leaves and divide the pecan mix among the leaves. Top with sliced red pepper, avocado, alfalfa sprouts and drizzle lime juice on top and sprinkle with sea salt.

Fold the top and bottom parts then roll up the sided.

Slice the wrap in two, if desired and serve immediately. Enjoy!

Nutritional Information per Serving:

Calories: 692; Total Fat: 47.9 g; Net Carbs: 11.2 g; Dietary Fiber: 16 g; Sugars: 6 g; Protein: 15.2 g; Cholesterol: 0 mg; Sodium: 264 mg

62.   Healthy Chickpea Veggie Sauté

Yield: 4 Servings
Total Time: 12 Minutes
Prep Time: 5 Minutes
Cook Time: 7 Minutes

Ingredients

- 3 tablespoons extra virgin olive oil
- 2 cups artichoke hearts
- 2 cups cooked chickpeas
- 1 tablespoon minced garlic
- 1 teaspoon coriander
- 2 teaspoons turmeric
- 1 teaspoon fenugreek seeds
- 1 teaspoon shaved ginger
- ½ teaspoon sea salt
- ½ teaspoon pepper

Directions

Heat a cast iron over medium high heat.

In a bowl, mix together olive oil, artichoke hearts, chickpeas and seasoning; toss into the hot skillet for about 6 minutes or until chickpeas are browned. Serve drizzled with fresh lemon juice.

Nutrition Information per Serving:

Calories: 314; Total Fat: 13.2 g; Net Carbs: 26 g; Dietary Fiber: 15.9 g; Sugars: 5.7 g Protein: 13 g; Cholesterol: 0 mg; Sodium: 395 mg

63.   Chicken Cacciatore with Brown Rice

Yield: 6 Servings
Total Time: 1 Hour 30 Minutes
Prep Time: 25 Minutes
Cook Time: 1 Hour 5 Minutes

Ingredients

- 6 (150g) chicken thighs, skinless
- 300g brown mushrooms, sliced
- 2 tablespoons olive oil
- 1/4 cup kalamata olives, pitted
- 200g cherry tomatoes
- 1 cup homemade chicken stock
- 1/2 cup balsamic vinegar
- 1 carrot, peeled, chopped
- 1 yellow capsicum, chopped
- 1 red onion, thinly sliced
- 1 red capsicum, chopped
- 4 garlic cloves, chopped
- 4 ripe tomatoes, chopped
- 2 tablespoons chopped fresh oregano
- 3 cups cooked brown rice

Directions

Sprinkle chicken with salt and pepper; heat oil in a large skillet over medium high heat and then cook in chicken for about 3 minutes per side. Transfer to a dish and keep warm. Add the mushrooms to the skillet and cook for about 4 minutes or until tender; transfer to a large bowl and the remaining oil to the skillet. Sauté in the red onions for about 2 minutes or until fragrant and tender. Stir in garlic and chopped tomatoes for about 4 minutes or until tender. Stir in carrots and capsicum for about 2 minutes and then add in vinegar. Cook for about 5 minutes or until liquid is reduced by half.

Return the mushroom and chicken to the pan and stir in olives, cherry tomatoes, grape tomatoes and stock and bring the mixture to a gentle boil. Lower heat and cook, covered, for about 20 minutes. Stir in chopped oregano.

Serve the chicken cacciatore with cooked brown rice.

Nutritional Information per Serving:

Calories: 498; Total Fat: 17.2 g; Net Carbs: 28.4 g; Dietary Fiber: 4.4 g; Sugars: 4.9 g; Protein: 49.3 g; Cholesterol: 134 mg; Sodium: 326 mg

64. Tasty Lemon Salmon Bake

Yield: 4 Servings
Total Time: 45 Minutes
Prep Time: 10 Minutes
Cook Time: 35 Minutes

Ingredients

- 4 (150g each) salmon fillets
- 1 bunch asparagus, trimmed
- 4 cups (600g) baby potatoes, diced
- 250g cherry tomatoes, diced
- 2 tablespoons extra-virgin olive oil
- 2 lemons, plus lemon zest to serve
- 8 sprigs fresh lemon thyme
- ¼ teaspoon sea salt

Directions

Preheat your oven to 400 degrees and line a greased baking tray with baking paper.

On the prepared tray, toss together lemon juice, potatoes, half of thyme, sea salt, lemon wedges and two teaspoons of oil until well coated.

Roast for about 15 minutes and then add in tomatoes; continue cooking for another 10 minutes.

Place the asparagus and salmon over the veggies and drizzle with the remaining oil.

Continue roasting for another 8 minutes.

Serve topped with lemon zest and thyme. Enjoy!

Nutritional Information per Serving:

Calories: 413; Total Fat: 18.5 g; Net Carbs: 19.5 g; Dietary Fiber: 6.6 g; Sugars: 2.9 g; Protein: 40 g; Cholesterol: 78 mg; Sodium: 216 mg

65.   Lime Turkey Breast & Avocado Salad

Yield: 6 Servings
Total Time: 10 Minutes
Prep Time: 10 Minutes
Cook Time: N/A

Ingredients
For the salad:
- o 2 1/4 pounds skinless turkey breasts
- o 1/2 cup fresh lime juice
- o A pinch of sea salt
- o 1 red bell pepper, sliced thinly
- o 2 cups broccoli florets
- o 2 large carrots, grated
- o 2 cups chopped red cabbage
- o 2 cups kale, chopped
- o 1 cup walnuts
- o 2 avocados, diced
- o 1/2 cup chopped parsley
- o 1 tablespoon sesame seeds

For the dressing:
- o 1/2 cup lemon juice, fresh
- o 1/3 cup grape seed oil
- o 2 teaspoons whole grain mustard
- o 1 tablespoon grated fresh ginger
- o 1/4 teaspoon sea salt
- o 1 tablespoon raw honey

Directions

In a small dish, mix lime juice, and salt; spread over the turkey and grill on a preheated charcoal grill for about 8 minutes per side or until cooked to your liking.

In a small bowl, whisk together all the dressing ingredients until well blended; set aside.

In a large bowl, combine kale, cabbage, broccoli, bell pepper, and carrots; pour over the dressing and toss until well coated.

Toss in walnuts, avocado, and parsley and sesame seeds until well combined.

Divide among serving bowls and top each with the grilled turkey and enjoy!

Nutritional Information per Serving:

Calories: 659; Total Fat: 37.8 g; Net Carbs: 14.2 g; Dietary Fiber: 9.1 g; Sugars: 7.6 g; Protein: 59.8 g; Cholesterol: 149 mg; Sodium: 209 mg

66.   Prawns Served with Whole-Wheat Bread

Yield: 6 Servings
Total Time: 25 Minutes
Prep Time: 15 Minutes
Cook Time: 10 Minutes

Ingredients

- o 1kg raw prawns, peeled, deveined
- o 4 shallots, finely chopped
- o 1/3 cup olive oil
- o 4 garlic cloves, finely chopped
- o 1/2 teaspoon fennel seeds
- o 2 tablespoon fresh flat-leaf parsley, chopped
- o 2 lemons, juiced
- o 1 tablespoon fresh lemon zest
- o 6 slices whole-wheat bread

Directions

Heat olive oil in a skillet set over medium heat; stir in shallots and fennel seedsand cook, stirring, for about 2 minutes or until shallot softens.

Stir in paprika, garlic and prawns and then season with salt. Cook for about 4 minutes or until prawns are cooked through.

Remove the skillet from heat and stir in parsley, lemon zest, and fresh lemon juice. Serve the prawns with sauce with the whole-wheat bread slices. Enjoy!

Nutritional Information per Serving:

Calories: 372; Total Fat: 15.1 g; Net Carbs: 15.5 g; Dietary Fiber: 2.4 g; Sugars: 3.6 g; Protein: 40.6 g; Cholesterol: 337 mg; Sodium: 525 mg

67. Chicken & Buckwheat Dinner Dish

Yield: 8 Servings
Total Time: 40 Minutes
Prep Time: 20 Minutes
Cook Time: 20 Minutes

Ingredients:
- 1 cup fresh lemon juice
- 2 teaspoons ground turmeric
- 2 tablespoons extra-virgin olive oil
- 8 (120g each) chicken breasts, skinless, boneless
- 2 cups chopped kale
- 1 tablespoon chopped ginger
- 2 large red onions, sliced
- 1 cup buckwheat

For the salsa
- 2 large tomatoes, finely chopped
- 2 tablespoons capers, finely chopped
- 1/2 cup fresh lemon juice
- ½ cup parsley, finely chopped
- 2 avocadoes, diced

Directions

Make salsa: mix avocado, chopped tomato, capers, chili, lemon juice, avocado, and parsley in a large bowl.

Preheat your oven to 450°F.

In a large bowl, mix lemon juice, 1 teaspoon turmeric, and a splash of extra virgin olive oil; add the chicken and stir to combine well. Marinate for about 10 minutes.

Set an ovenproof pan over medium heat and add the chicken; cook for about 4 minutes per side or until lightly browned. Transfer to the preheated oven and bake for about 10 minutes remove from the oven and

Remove the chicken from oven and keep warm.

In the meantime, steam kale in a steamer for about 5 minutes.

Fry ginger and red onion in a splash of extra virgin olive oil until tender; stir in kale and cook for about 1 minute.

Follow package instructions to cook buckwheat with the remaining turmeric.

Serve the buckwheat with chicken, veggies and salsa.

Nutritional Information per Serving:

Calories: 492; Total Fat: 23.5 g; Net Carbs: 23 g; Dietary Fiber: 8.4 g; sugars: 4.3 g; Protein: 41.2 g; Cholesterol: 107 mg; Sodium: 327 mg

68.   Lemon Grilled Fish with Salsa

Yield: 4 Servings
Total Time: 20 Minutes
Prep Time: 10 Minutes
Cook Time: 10 Minutes

Ingredients

- 4 (120g each) white fish fillets
- 2 bunches asparagus, ends removed
- 2 bunches baby broccoli, ends removed
- 1 red onion, finely chopped
- 1 avocado, diced
- 2 large cucumbers, diced
- 2 large tomatoes, finely chopped
- 2 tablespoons shredded mint leaves
- 2 tablespoons chopped capers
- 2 tablespoons lemon juice
- 1 teaspoon lemon zest
- 1 tablespoon olive oil
- 1/2 teaspoons salt

Directions

In a bowl, mix together oil, mint, capers, red onion, cucumber, avocado, and tomatoes; drizzle with half of lemon juice and season with salt and set aside.

In a small bowl, mix together the remaining lemon juice, lemon zest, pepper and salt; rub over the fish until well coated.

Heat the BBQ grill on medium high heat and spray the asparagus and broccoli with olive oil; season with salt and pepper; grill for about 2 minutes per side or until crisp and charred. Transfer to a plate and keep warm.

Drizzle fish with olive oil and grill for about 3 minutes per side or until cooked through and golden browned on both sides. Divide the asparagus and broccoli on serving plates and top each with the tomato mixture and grilled fish.

Nutritional Information per Serving:

Calories: 472; Total Fat: 25.6 g; Net Carbs: 12.6 g; Dietary Fiber: 7.7 g; Sugars: 7.5 g; Protein: 42.5 g; Cholesterol: 119 mg; Sodium: 548 mg

69. Pan-SearedTurkey with Orange Chimichurri

Yield: 3 Servings
Total Time: 5 Minutes
Prep Time: 5 Minutes
Cook Time: 5 Minutes

Ingredients

- 1 teaspoon finely grated orange zest
- 1 teaspoon dried oregano
- 1 small garlic clove, grated
- 2 teaspoon apple cider vinegar
- 1 tablespoon fresh orange juice
- 1/2 cup chopped fresh flat-leaf parsley leaves
- 1 1/2 pound skinless turkey breasts, quartered
- ¼ teaspoon sea salt
- 1/4 cup and 2 teaspoons extra virgin olive oil
- 4 cups arugula
- 2 bulbs fennel, shaved
- 2 tablespoons whole-grain mustard

Directions

Make chimichurri: In a medium bowl, combine orange zest, oregano and garlic. Mix in vinegar, orange juice and parsley and then slowly whisk in ¼ cup of olive oil until emulsified. Season with sea salt.

Sprinkle the steak with salt; heat the remaining olive oil in a large skillet and cook turkey over medium high heat for about 6 minutes per side or until browned. Remove from heat and let rest for at least 10 minutes.

Toss fennel, greens, turkey, mustard, sea salt and pepper until well combined.

Serve turkey with chimichurri and salad. Enjoy!

Nutritional Information per Serving:

Calories: 457; Total Fat: 27.5 g; Net Carbs: 2 g; Dietary Fiber: 0.8 g; Sugars: 1 g; Protein: 20.8 g; Cholesterol: 132 mg; Sodium: 195 mg

70. Coconut& Lemon Chicken Bake

Yield: 4 Servings
Total Time: 1 Hour 15 Minutes
Prep Time: 15 Minutes
Cook Time: 1 Hour

Ingredients

- 4 skinless chicken breasts
- 1 large eggplant, diced
- 1 butternut squash, diced
- 4 tablespoons gluten-free breadcrumb
- 3 tablespoons desiccated coconut
- 2 tablespoons extra-virgin olive oil
- 2 tablespoons freshly squeezed lemon juice
- 2 tablespoons red curry paste
- ¼ teaspoon sea salt
- ¼ teaspoon black pepper
- 300g cherry tomato
- lime wedges
- handful coriander, chopped

Directions

Preheat oven to 400ºF.

Toss together half of the olive oil, eggplant, and squash in a large bowl; spread out in a roasting pan and roast for about 30 minutes, turning once.

Mix bread crumbs, coconut, sea salt and pepper on a plate; drizzle the chicken with the remaining olive oil and fresh lemon juice and then press into the crumb mixture.

Stir curry paste and tomatoes in the roasted veggies and nestle chicken in the center of the veggies.

Bake in the oven for about 30 minutes or until chicken is cooked through. Serve garnished with lime wedges and coriander.

Nutritional Info per Serving:

Calories: 477; Total Fat: 22.7 g; Carbs: 19.8 g; Dietary Fiber: 4.3 g; Sugars: 5.2 g; Protein: 45.9 g; Cholesterol: 171 mg; Sodium: 586 mg

71.   Grilled Burritos with Cashew Crema

Yield: 4 Servings
Total Time: 20 Minutes
Prep Time: 10 Minutes
Cook Time: 10 Minutes

Ingredients

For Salsa Crema:
- 1 tablespoon lemon juice
- 1/2 cup raw walnuts
- 1/2 cup raw cashews
- 3/4 cup your favorite roasted salsa
- 3/4 cup Silk Cashew Milk

For Burritos:
- 4 whole wheat tortillas
- 3/4 cup cooked black beans
- 3/4 cup cooked brown rice
- 1/2 avocado, sliced
- Sea salt
- Chopped cilantro
- corn

Directions

In a blender, blend all cream ingredients until very smooth; set aside.

In a large bowl, combine cooked beans, rice, and salt; divide the mixture between the two tortillas and top with sliced avocado. Fold to enclose the filling and place them, seam side down, on a frying pan. Cook on medium low heat for about 5 minutes or until the tortillas are browned; flip over and cook the other side. Place the tortillas on serving plates and drizzle each with salsa crema. Serve garnished with chopped cilantro and corn.

Nutrition Information per Serving

Calories: 588; Total Fat: 16 g; Carbs: 77.5 g; Dietary Fiber: 12.6 g; Sugars: 3.3 g; Protein: 20.7 g Cholesterol: 0 mg; Sodium: 79 mg

72.   Spiced Lentils with Brown Rice

Yield: 3 Servings
Total Time: 5 Minutes
Prep Time: 5 Minutes
Cook Time: N/A

Ingredients

- 5 cups water
- 1 cup mixed lentils and split peas
- 3 tablespoons minced garlic
- 1 teaspoon turmeric
- 1 teaspoon cumin
- 1 teaspoon curry powder
- ½ teaspoon sea salt
- ½ cup brown rice
- 2 cups frozen veggies

Directions

Bring water to a rolling boil in a pot; add the lentils and split peas, garlic and spices and cook for about 50 minutes or until lentils are tender. Add frozen veggies to lentils and cook for 5 minutes more.

Meanwhile, boil rice in salted water until tender. Serve the lentil-veggie stew over rice.

Nutritional Information per Serving:

Calories: 330 Total Fat: 1.6 g; Carbs: 62 g; Dietary Fiber: 20 g; Sugars: 3.9 g; Protein: 17.4 g; Cholesterol: 0 mg; Sodium: 281 mg

73.   Chicken & Buckwheat Salad

Yield: 8 Servings
Total Time: 40 Minutes
Prep Time: 20 Minutes
Cook Time: 20 Minutes

Ingredients:
- 1 cup fresh lemon juice
- 2 teaspoons ground turmeric
- 2 tablespoons extra-virgin olive oil
- 8 (120g each) chicken breasts, skinless, boneless
- 2 cups chopped kale
- 1 tablespoon chopped ginger
- 2 large red onions, sliced
- 1 cup buckwheat

For the salsa
- 2 large tomatoes, finely chopped
- 2 tablespoons capers, finely chopped
- 1/2 cup fresh lemon juice
- ½ cup parsley, finely chopped
- 2 avocadoes, diced

Directions

Make salsa: mix avocado, chopped tomato, capers, lemon juice, avocado, and parsley in a large bowl.

Preheat your oven to 450°F.

In a large bowl, mix lemon juice, 1 teaspoon turmeric, and a splash of extra virgin olive oil; add the chicken and stir to combine well. Marinate for about 10 minutes.

Set an ovenproof pan over medium heat and add the chicken; cook for about 4 minutes per side or until lightly browned. Transfer to the preheated oven and bake for about 10 minutes remove from the oven and

Remove the chicken from oven and keep warm.

In the meantime, steam kale in a steamer for about 5 minutes.

Fry ginger and red onion in a splash of extra virgin olive oil until tender; stir in kale and cook for about 1 minute.

Follow package instructions to cook buckwheat with the remaining turmeric.

Serve the buckwheat with chicken, veggies and salsa.

Nutritional Information per Serving:

Calories: 492; Total Fat: 23.5 g; Net Carbs: 23 g; Dietary Fiber: 8.4 g; sugars: 4.3 g; Protein: 41.2 g; Cholesterol: 107 mg; Sodium: 327 mg

74. Mushroom Marinara with Buckwheat Pasta

Yield: 2 Servings
Total Time: 45 Minutes
Prep Time: 10 Minutes
Cook Time: 35 Minutes

Ingredients:

- 1/2 cup water
- ½ cup chopped red onion
- 3-4 cups sliced mushrooms
- 2 garlic cloves, minced
- 1/2 teaspoon fennel seeds
- 1 teaspoon dried thyme
- 1 teaspoon dried oregano
- 1 teaspoon dried basil
- 4 cups tomato sauce
- 2 cups chopped tomatoes
- 1 pound whole-wheat pasta

Directions:

Cook red onions in water for about 2 minutes; stir in mushrooms and garlic and cook for about 5 minutes or until mushrooms are lightly browned and onion is tender.

Stir in fennels seeds, thyme, oregano, basil, tomato sauce and tomato and simmer for about 30 minutes.

Follow package instructions to cook pasta until tender; drain and serve topped with the mushroom sauce. Enjoy!

Nutrition Information per Serving

Calories: 194; Total Fat: 1.8 g; Carbs: 41.6 g; Dietary Fiber: 12 g; Sugars: 28.7 g; Protein: 12.1 g Cholesterol: 0 mg; Sodium: 2587 mg

75.   Delicious Sweet Potato & Bean Curry

Yield: 4-6 Servings
Total Time: 1 Hour 55 Minutes
Prep Time: 20 Minutes
Cook Time: 1 hour 35 Minutes

Ingredients

- 2 sweet potatoes, peeled and chopped
- 1 can (14 ounces) cannellini beans
- 1 can (14 ounces) tomatoes
- Olive oil
- 1 yellow onion, chopped
- 1 yellow pepper, chopped
- 2 red bell peppers, chopped
- 1 bunch fresh coriander, finely chopped
- 1 tablespoon cumin powder
- 1 teaspoon smoked paprika
- 2 teaspoons cinnamon powder

Directions

Preheat your oven to 350 degrees F.

Arrange the sweet potato in a roasting tray and drizzle with olive oil. Toss with a pinch each of cumin, cinnamon and paprika.

Spread the potatoes in one layer and roast for about 40 minutes until soft

Add 1 tablespoon of oil in a pan and sauté the onion, peppers, coriander, chili and all the remaining spices.

Cook on low for 15 minutes, stirring so the veggies don't stick to the pan.

Stir in the beans together with the liquid and the tomatoes. Stir well to combine and add a splash of water, if needed. Simmer for half an hour then stir in the baked sweet potatoes.

Serve over a bed of steamed rice with sliced avocado on the side, if desired.

Nutritional Information per Serving:

Calories: 358; Total Fat: 8.6 g; Carbs: 56.9 g; Dietary Fiber: 13.4g; Sugars: 6.2 g; Protein: 12.4 g; Cholesterol: 16 mg; Sodium: 30 mg

76.   Veggie Noodles in Coconut Sauce

Yield: 2 Servings
Total Time: 50 Minutes
Prep Time: 20 Minutes
Cook Time: 30 Minutes

Ingredients

- 2 green zucchini
- 2 yellow zucchini
- 7 ounces mangetout or fresh peas
- 2 corn cobs
- 1 handful of fresh mixed herbs, chopped

For the sauce:

- 1 banana shallot, chopped
- 2 teaspoons ground turmeric
- 1 clove garlic, finely chopped
- ½ teaspoon ginger paste
- 10 ounces coconut water
- 7 ounces coconut milk
- 1 teaspoon hot curry powder
- 4 ounces desiccated coconut, unsweetened
- Juice of 1 lime

Directions

Start by making the sauce

Combine all the sauce ingredients in your food processor and pulse until perfectly smooth.

Using a spiralizer or julienne peeler, cut the carrot and zucchini into long and thin noodles. Combine with the rest of the veggies in a bowl. For the mangetout, slice it diagonally.

Steam the veggies in the microwave, if desired and drizzle with the spicy coconut sauce.

Garnish with the mixed herbs, cover and let marinate for half an hour.

Serve with lime wedges.

Nutritional Information per Serving:

Calories: 598; Total Fat: 36.2 g; Carbs: 53.4 g; Dietary Fiber: 16.8g; Sugars: 25.6 g; Protein: 18.8 g; Cholesterol: 28 mg; Sodium: 42 mg

77. Delicious Chicken Curry

Yield: 1 Serving
Total Time: 30 Minutes
Prep Time: 10 Minutes
Cook Time: 20 Minutes

Ingredients

- 100 grams chicken, diced
- ¼ cup chicken broth
- Pinch of turmeric
- Dash of onion powder
- 1 tablespoon minced red onion
- Pinch of garlic powder
- ¼ teaspoon curry powder
- Pinch of sea salt
- Raw honey, optional

Directions

In a small saucepan, stir spices in chicken broth until dissolved; stir in chicken, garlic, onion, and honey and cook until chicken is cooked through and liquid is reduced by half. Serve hot.

Nutritional Information per Serving:

Calories: 170; Total Fat: 3.5 g; Carbs: 2.3 g; Dietary Fiber: 0.6 g; Sugars: 0.8 g; Protein: 30.5 g; Cholesterol: 77 mg; Sodium: 255 mg

78.   Grilled Chicken Breast with Nutty Greek Yogurt

Yield: 3 Servings
Total Time: 2 Hours 10 Minutes
Prep Time: 2 Hours
Cook Time: 10 Minutes

Ingredients

For the Grilled Chicken:
- 3 boneless chicken breast halves, skinned
- 1 clove garlic, minced
- 1 tablespoon fresh lemon juice, freshly squeezed
- 1 tablespoon extra-virgin olive oil
- 1 teaspoon dried oregano
- ¼ teaspoon sea salt

For the yogurt:
- 1 cup nonfat Greek yogurt
- 1/4 cup fresh lime juice
- 1 clove garlic, minced
- 1 teaspoon fresh dill, minced
- ½ cup cucumber, very thinly sliced or shredded
- ½ cup pistachios, shelled and chopped, (divide into 2)

Directions

Use a sharp knife to gently slice through the thickest part of the chicken breast with cutting all the way through so you are able to open it up like a book. Do this for the other two halves. Marinate the chicken with the remaining chicken ingredients in a large bowl. Cover with cling wrap and set in the fridge for 1 ½ to 2 hours.

Preheat your grill to medium-high heat. Take out the chicken from the marinade. Lightly grease your grill rack then place the breasts on top. Cook for about 3 minutes on each side or until done to desire.

Meanwhile, combine all the yogurt ingredients in a medium bowl. Remember to set aside one half of the pistachios.

To serve, serve each breast on a large plate. Place a dollop of the nutty yogurt on the side and top the chicken with the remaining pistachios. Enjoy!

Nutritional Information per Serving:

Calories: 318; Total Fat: 13g; Carbs: 8g; Dietary Fiber: 4g; Protein: 37g; Cholesterol: 38mg; Sodium: 468mg

79.   Grilled Lemon Chicken Salad

Yield: 8 Servings
Total Time: 25 Minutes
Prep Time: 10 Minutes
Cook Time: 15 Minutes

Ingredients
For the dressing
- 1/2 cup groundnut oil
- 1 teaspoon raw honey
- 3 tablespoons fresh lemon juice
- 2 tablespoons orange juice
- ½ teaspoon finely grated orange zest
- 1 teaspoon Dijon mustard
- 1 garlic clove, crushed
- 2 teaspoons freshly grated ginger

For the salad
- 1kg skinless boneless chicken breasts
- 4 tablespoons fresh lemon juice
- A pinch of sea salt
- 2 cups chopped watercress
- 4 cups chopped lettuce
- 2 large heads of chicory, chopped
- 3 oranges, peeled, segmented, and deseeded

Directions
Combine all salad ingredients and chill for at least 1 hour.

Meanwhile, in a small bowl, whisk together lemon juice, sea salt and pepper until well combined; add in chicken breasts and toss to coat well. Place on a preheated charcoal grill and cook for about 8 minutes per side or until cooked through and golden brown.

In a jar, combine all dressing ingredients and shake to mix well. Chill in the refrigerator for at least 2 days before using.

Serve the salad drizzled with the dressing and mix to coat well. Top each serving with grilled chicken. Enjoy!

80. Chicken with Healthy Almond & Pistachio Pesto

Yield: 4 Servings
Total Time: 15 Minutes
Prep Time: 10 Minutes
Cook Time: 5 Minutes

Ingredients

- 4 (180g) chicken breasts
- 1 tablespoon extra-virgin olive oil
- 1 cup baby Spinach
- 1 cup rocket
- 1 cup halved cherry tomatoes

Almond & Pistachio pesto

- 1/2 cup extra-virgin olive oil
- 1/3 cup toasted pistachios
- 1/3 cup toasted almonds
- 1/4 cup fresh lime juice
- 1 red onion, chopped
- 1/4 cup basil leaves
- 1/2 cup mint leaves
- 1 cup baby rocket

Directions

In a food processor, process together fresh lime juice, pistachios, garlic, basil, mint, rocket, and toasted almonds until very smooth; add in oil, salt and pepper and continue pulsing until very smooth. Set aside.

Preheat the BBQ grill on medium heat and then brush the chicken with oil; season with salt and pepper.

Grill for about 3 minutes per side or until cooked to your desire. Transfer to a plate and cover with a plastic wrap.

Slice the chicken and divide among the serving plates; top each serving with spinach and tomatoes and season with salt and pepper.

Serve with the creamy almond and pistachio pesto.

Nutritional Information per Serving:

Calories: 591; Total Fat: 35.3 g; Net Carbs: 7 g; Dietary Fiber: 3.9 g; Sugars: 3.6 g; Protein: 59 g; Cholesterol: 161 mg; Sodium: 161 mg

81.   Grilled Chicken Salad with Macadamia Dressing

Yield: 3 Servings
Total Time: 15 Minutes
Prep Time: 10 Minutes
Cook Time: 5 Minutes

Ingredients
For the Dressing
- 2 tablespoons freshly squeezed orange juice
- 2 tablespoons freshly squeezed lemon juice
- 3 tablespoons extra-virgin olive oil
- 1/2 teaspoon raw honey
- 1 teaspoon raw apple-cider vinegar
- 4 fresh sliced basil leaves
- 1 1/2 tablespoons chopped fresh parsley
- 1 1/2 tablespoons chopped fresh dill
- 1/4 cup toasted and chopped macadamia nuts
- ¼ teaspoon coarse salt

For the Salad
- 3/4 pound grilled chicken
- 1 cup asparagus, trimmed
- 1/2 cup carrots, scrubbed
- 1/4 pound green beans, trimmed
- 1/2 large fennel bulb, cut into 1/2-inch slices
- ½ tsp. coarse salt

Directions

In a bowl, whisk together the dressing ingredients and season with salt; set aside.

Steam veggies in steamer set over a saucepan of boiling water for about 5 minutes or until crisp tender.

Half the steamed carrots and asparagus spears lengthwise.

Arrange the veggies on a serving platter and sprinkle with salt; Top with grilled chicken and drizzle with the dressing and garnish with herbs.

Macros Breakdown:

Calories: 515; Fat: 35.8 g; Carbs: 13.8 g; Dietary Fiber: 7.2 g; Sugars: 2.2 g; Protein: 39.3 g; Cholesterol: 255 mg; Sodium: 581 mg

82.   Coconut Lentil Soup with Brown Rice

Yield: 6 Servings
Total Time: 45 Minutes
Prep Time: 15 Minutes
Cook Time: 30 Minutes

Ingredients

- 6 cups vegetable broth
- 1 red onion, diced
- 2 cups red lentils
- 2 kaffir lime leaves
- 1 tablespoon chopped fresh garlic
- 1 tablespoon grated fresh ginger
- 1 tablespoon lemongrass paste
- 1 cup coconut milk
- 2 cups diced butternut squash
- 1 tablespoon curry powder
- a pinch of sea salt
- 1 teaspoon raw honey
- 1 cup hot cooked brown rice
- sliced green onions
- fresh cilantro

Directions

In a large pot, mix together lentils, broth and red onion and bring to a gentle boil.

Cover and let the mixture cook on medium heat until lentils are tender and then stir in squash, coconut milk, lemongrass paste, ginger, garlic, kaffir lime leaves, curry powder, and salt.

Continue cooking for another 10 minutes and then stir in stevia.

Serve the soup over cooked brown rice; garnish with green onions and cilantro and serve.

Nutritional Information per Serving:

Calories: 512; Total Fat: 12.7 g; Carbs: 75.8 g; Dietary Fiber: 23.4 g; Sugars: 5.3 g; Protein: 25.7 g; Cholesterol: 0 mg; Sodium: 822 mg

83.   Lemony Salmon with Crunchy Slaw

Yield: 4 Servings
Total Time: 25 Minutes
Prep Time: 15 Minutes
Cook Time: 10 Minutes

Ingredients

- 4 x 150g salmon
- 2 tablespoons olive oil
- 4 cups thinly sliced purple cabbage
- 2 tablespoons raw honey
- 1/2 cup fresh lime juice
- 1 teaspoon lime zest
- 2 spring onions, chopped
- 1 yellow capsicum, thinly sliced
- 200g seedless white grapes, halved
- 1/2 cup fresh mint leaves
- 1 cup fresh coriander leaves
- 1 cup chopped toasted macadamias

Directions

Whisk together two tablespoons of fresh lime juice and sea salt in a small bowl. Add in the salmon and turn until well coated with the mixture.

Heat half oil in a skillet over medium heat; place in salmon and cook for about 5 minutes or until the skin is crisp; turn over to cook the other side for about 3 minutes or until cooked through.

In the meantime, whisk together the remaining lime juice, raw honey, lime zest, salt, pepper and the remaining oil until well blended; add in grapes, cabbage, spring onions, capsicum, mint and coriander.

Dry toast the cashew nuts in a pan until fragrant and golden brown. Add to the cabbage slaw and toss to combine well.

Divide the cabbage slaw among serving plates and top each serving with salmon serve right away!

Nutritional Information per Serving:

Calories: 600; Total Fat: 21 g; Net Carbs: 24.2 g; Dietary Fiber: 6.6 g; Sugars: 21.4 g; Protein: 33.8 g; Cholesterol: 66 mg; Sodium: 90 mg

84. Grilled Salmon with Creamy Salsa

Yield: 4 Servings
Total Time: 30 Minutes
Prep Time: 20 Minutes
Cook Time: 10 Minutes

Ingredients

- 4 (120g each) skinless salmon fillets
- 1 teaspoon dried oregano
- 1 teaspoon onion powder
- 1 teaspoon ground coriander
- 1 tablespoon extra-virgin olive oil
- 2 cups chopped lettuce

Avocado-Mango Salsa

- 1 red onion, chopped
- 1 cucumber, chopped
- 1 tomato
- 1 avocado, diced
- 1 mango, diced
- 2 tablespoons lime juice
- 1 cup chopped coriander

Directions

In a bowl, mix together onion powder, coriander, and oil until well combined; add in salmon and turn until well coated; sprinkle with salt and pepper.

Preheat the grill on medium high and grill the fish for about 3 minutes per side or until cooked to your liking. Wrap in foil and let set for at least 5 minutes.

In the meantime, in a bowl, mix together avocado, mango, red onion, cucumber, coriander, and fresh lime juice until well combined.

Divide lettuce on serving plates and top each with the grilled salmon and salsa. Serve right away.

Nutritional Information per Serving:

Calories: 383; Total Fat: 21.5 g; Net Carbs: 19.5 g; Dietary Fiber: 6.7 g; Sugars: 15.4 g; Protein: 26.5 g; Cholesterol: 53 mg; Sodium: 65 mg

85.   BBQ Chicken Breast Salad

Yield: 4 Servings
Total Time: 30 Minutes
Prep Time: 20 Minutes
Cook Time: 10 Minutes

Ingredients

- 600g skinless chicken breasts
- 1 cup green salad
- 2 heads baby lettuce
- 2 radishes, sliced
- 1 nectarine, pitted and sliced
- 1 carrot, peeled, shaved
- 3 baby cucumbers, shaved
- 1 avocado
- 1 cup fresh coriander leaves
- 1 cup small fresh mint leaves

Dressing

- 4 tablespoons olive oil, divided
- 1/4 cup fresh lime juice
- 1 tablespoon grated peeled ginger
- 2 tablespoons chopped shallot
- Sea salt

Directions

Preheat your BBQ grill on medium high.

In a blender, blend together shallot, fish sauce, three tablespoons of olive oil, lime juice, ginger and raw honey until very smooth; set aside.

Brush the remaining oil over the chicken and sprinkle with salt; barbecue the meat for about 4 minutes per side or until cooked through.

Transfer the chicken to a chopping board and slice into small pieces.

Divide salad mix, lettuce leaves, radishes, avocado, cucumbers, nectarine, carrots, coriander, and mint on serving plates and drizzle with the dressing; toss to coat well. Top each serving with sliced chicken and serve with the remaining dressing. Enjoy!

Nutritional Information per Serving:

Calories: 561; Total Fat: 33.4 g; Net Carbs: 10.7 g; Dietary Fiber: 6.9 g; Sugars: 6 g; Protein: 49.4 g; Cholesterol: 134 mg; Sodium: 815 mg

86.   Grilled Chicken Breast with Nutty Pesto

Yield: 4 Servings
Total Time: 15 Minutes
Prep Time: 10 Minutes
Cook Time: 5 Minutes

Ingredients

- 4 (180g) skinless chicken breasks
- 1 tablespoon extra-virgin olive oil
- 1 cup baby Spinach
- 1 cup rocket
- 1 cup halved cherry tomatoes
- **Nutty Pesto**
- 1/2 cup extra-virgin olive oil
- 1/3 cup toasted pistachios
- 1/3 cup toasted almonds
- 1/4 cup fresh lime juice
- 1 red onion, chopped
- 1/4 cup basil leaves
- 1/2 cup mint leaves
- 1 cup baby rocket

Directions

In a food processor, process together fresh lime juice, pistachios, garlic, basil, mint, rocket, and toasted almonds until very smooth; add in oil, salt and pepper and continue pulsing until very smooth. Set aside.

Preheat the BBQ grill on medium heat and then brush the chicken with oil; season with salt. Grill for about 3 minutes per side or until cooked to your desire. Transfer to a plate and cover with a plastic wrap.

Slice the chicken breasts and divide among the serving plates; top each serving with spinach and tomatoes and season with salt and pepper.

Serve with the creamy almond and pistachio pesto.

Nutritional Information per Serving:

Calories: 591; Total Fat: 35.3 g; Net Carbs: 7 g; Dietary Fiber: 3.9 g; Sugars: 3.6 g; Protein: 59 g; Cholesterol: 161 mg; Sodium: 161 mg

87.   Turkey Patty Salad with Lemony Tahini Sauce

Yield: 8 Servings
Total Time: 26 Minutes
Prep Time: 10 Minutes
Cook Time: 16 Minutes

Ingredients

- 2 pounds ground turkey
- 3/4 teaspoon ground ginger
- 1 teaspoon dried sage
- 1/2 teaspoons salt
- 4 cups of green salad for serving

Low Carb Lemon Tahini Sauce

- 4 tablespoons lemon juice
- ½ cup organic tahini
- 1 tablespoon extra-virgin olive oil
- 2 cloves garlic
- ⅓ cup water
- A pinch sea salt

Directions

Prepare Tahini: in a blender, blend together all ingredients until very smooth. Refrigerate until ready to use.

Mix together ground turkey, sage, ginger, and salt in a bowl until well blended. Form patties from the mixture and place on a plate.

Heat olive oil in a skillet over medium high heat and fry the patties for about 8 minutes per side or until no longer pink in the inside and browned on the outside.

Serve the turkey patties with green salad drizzled with lemon tahini.

Nutritional Information per Serving:

Calories: 333; Total Fat: 22.4 g; Carbs: 4.4 g; Dietary Fiber: 1.8 g; Sugars: 0.5 g; Protein: 34 g; Cholesterol: 116 mg; Sodium: 308 mg

88.   Stir-Fried Chicken & Green Bean

Yield: 4 Servings
Total Time: 20 Minutes
Prep Time: 5 Minutes
Cook Time: 15 Minutes

Ingredients

- 500g ground chicken
- 2 cups sliced green beans
- 1 cup freshly squeezed lemon juice
- 1 tablespoon oyster sauce
- 1/3 cup chopped mint leaves
- 1 cup fresh coriander sprigs
- 3 garlic cloves, sliced
- Steamed veggies

Directions

Heat oil in a skillet set over medium heat; sauté garlic for about 2 minutes or until fragrant; transfer to a plate and add chicken to the skillet.

Fry for about 5 minutes or until browned.

Add in seasoning and cook for one minute; stir in lemon juice and oyster sauce. Simmer for about 10 minutes or until the mixture in thick.

Stir in beans and cook for about 2 minutes or until crisp. Stir in mint and coriander and serve sprinkled with garlic.

Serve over a bowl of steamed veggies.

Nutritional Information per Serving:

Calories: 280; Total Fat: 8.4 g; Carbs: 8.2 g; Dietary Fiber: 3.1 g; Sugars: 2.1 g; Protein: 40.3 g; Cholesterol: 112 mg; Sodium: 130 mg

89.   Stir-Fried Veggies with Seared Lemon Chicken

Yield: 3- 4 Servings
Total Time: 25 Minutes
Prep Time: 15 Minutes
Cook Time: 10 Minutes

Ingredients for

- 1 pound skinless chicken breasts
- ¼ cup fresh lemon juice
- 1 tablespoon lemon zest
- 3 tablespoon extra-virgin olive oil
- 1 cup chopped red onion
- 4 cloves garlic, minced
- 2 cups cremini mushrooms, diced
- 3 medium zucchinis

- 1 green pepper bell
- 1 red pepper bell
- 1 ½ cups unsweetened almond milk
- ¼ tablespoon ginger
- ½ tablespoon curry powder
- A pinch of sea salt

Directions

Rub the chicken with lemon juice and dust with lemon zest, cayenne pepper, and sea salt; heat half of the olive oil in a skillet set over medium heat and sear in the meat for about 6 minutes per side or until cooked through and golden browned on the outside.

Keep the meat warm wrapped in a foil.

Dice zucchinis, bell peppers, and beans in bite-size pieces. Heat oil in a pan and fry the red onion and garlic; add in mushrooms, zucchini, and bell peppers; fry for 3 minutes more.

Stir in milk and cook for a few minutes.

Season with ginger, curry powder, and salt. Serve topped with sliced chicken.

Nutritional Information Per Serving:

Calories: 381; Total Fat: 19.4 g; Carbs: 14.7 g; Dietary Fiber: 4 g; Sugars: 6.6 g; Protein: 37.7 g; Cholesterol: 101 mg; Sodium: 212 mg

90.   Creamy Lemon Corn Snack

Yield: 4 Servings
Total Time: 20 Minutes
Prep Time: 10 Minutes
Cook Time: 10 Minutes

Ingredients

- 2 cup corn kernels
- 2 tablespoons chopped red bell pepper
- 2 tablespoons chopped cilantro
- ½ teaspoon cumin seeds
- 1 teaspoon olive oil
- 2 tablespoons coconut cream
- 2 tablespoons lemon juice
- ½ teaspoon salt

Directions

Lightly grease a heavy pan with oil and then fry in corn kernels for about 5 minutes or until lightly browned.

Remove from heat and stir in cumin seed powder, salt, red bell pepper, cilantro, coconut cream, and lemon juice.

Mix to combine well and serve warm. Enjoy!

Nutritional Information per Serving:

Calories: 115; Total Fat: 4 g; Net Carbs: 16.7 g; Dietary Fiber: 3.1 g; Sugars: 5.9 g; Protein: 3.3 g; Cholesterol: 0 mg; Sodium: 321 mg

91.   Healthy Berry & Nut Bars

Yield: 8 Servings
Total Time: 30 Minutes
Prep Time: 10 Minutes
Cook Time: 20 Minutes

Ingredients:

- 1 cup goji berries
- 1 cup pumpkin seeds
- 1 cup almonds
- 1 cup walnuts
- 6 dates

- ½ cups cocoa nibs
- ½ cup agave
- 2 tablespoons coconut flour
- 1 teaspoon vanilla
- ½ teaspoon sea salt

Directions:

Preheat oven to 350°F.

In a food processor, grind pumpkin seeds, almonds, and walnuts until roughly chopped.
Add dates and continue processing until roughly chopped.

Transfer the mixture to a large bowl and stir in the remaining ingredients. Spread the mixture into an

8×8-inch baking dish and bake for about 20 minutes.

Remove from oven and let cool before cutting into bars. Enjoy!

Nutritional Information per Serving:

Calories: 396; Total Fat: 25.1 g; Carbs: 36.4 g; Dietary Fiber: 6.9 g; Sugars: 26.2 g; Protein: 11.7 g; Cholesterol: 0 mg; Sodium: 121 mg

92.   Toasted Almonds & Seed Mix

Yield: 3 Servings
Total Time: 20 Minutes
Prep Time: 10 Minutes
Cook Time: 10 Minutes

Ingredients

- 2 tablespoons olive oil
- 1/2 cup sunflower seeds
- 1/2 cup pumpkin seeds
- 1 cup almonds

- 1 tablespoon crushed fennel seeds
- 1 tablespoon ground cumin
- ½ teaspoon sea salt

Directions

Heat oil in a skillet set over medium heat; stir in chili paste and fennel seeds and then add in seeds and almonds; sauté for about 5 minutes and then stir in cumin and salt.
Remove from heat and let cool before serving.

Nutritional Information per Serving:

Calories: 462; Total Fat: 6.6 g; Net Carbs: 9.8 g; Dietary Fiber: 6.5 g; Sugars: 3.3 g; Protein: 14.9 g; Cholesterol: 1 mg; Sodium: 278 mg

93.   Healthy Superfood Raw Bars

Yield: 15 Servings (30 Bars)
Total Time: 10 Minutes
Prep Time: 15 Minutes
Cook Time: 5 Minutes

Ingredients

- 1 cup toasted pistachios
- 1 cup goji berries
- 1/2 cup roasted almonds
- 2 tablespoons chia seeds
- 1 cup coconut flakes, toasted
- 1/3 cup ginger
- 1 tablespoon raw cacao nibs
- 1 tablespoon coconut oil
- 300g chopped dark chocolate
- Pinch of sea salt

Directions

Prepare a baking pan by greasing and lining with baking paper.

In a large bowl, combine 1/2 cup of pistachios, 1/2 cup of coconut flakes, goji berries, almond, chia pieces, and ginger until well mixed.

In another bowl, stir together cacao nibs, the remaining pistachios and coconut flakes, and more goji berries.

In a saucepan, stir together oil, chocolate and salt until chocolate is melted. Pour the chocolate mixture into the pistachio mixture and stir until well coated; transfer to the pan and sprinkle with the cacao mixture. Refrigerate for at least 4 hours or until firm.

Cut into 24 squares and serve, storing the rest in the refrigerator for up two weeks.

Nutritional Information per Serving:

Calories: 246; Total Fat: 13.7 g; Net Carbs: 23.6 g; Dietary Fiber: 4.8 g; Sugars: 20.6 g; Protein: 4.3 g; Cholesterol: 5 mg; Sodium: 55 mg

94.   Avocado & Pea Dip with Carrots

Yield: 3 Servings
Total Time: 10 Minutes
Prep Time: 10 Minutes
Cook Time: N/A

Ingredients

- o 1 avocado, peeled and seed removed
- o 1 1/2 cups steamed snow peas
- o 2 tablespoons lime juice
- o I clove of garlic, diced
- o 6 carrots to serve

Directions

Combine together all ingredients in a blender and blend until very smooth. Serve with fresh carrots.

Nutritional Information per Serving:

Calories: 230; Total Fat: 12.2 g; Net Carbs: 16.4 g; Dietary Fiber: 10 g; Sugars: 10 g; Protein: 5.2 g; Cholesterol: 0 mg; Sodium: 92 mg

95. Tangy Carrot & Parsnips French Fries

Yield: 6 Servings
Total Time: 35 Minutes
Prep Time: 15 Minutes
Cook Time: 20 Minutes

Ingredients

- 6 large carrots
- 3 large parsnips
- 2 tablespoons extra virgin olive oil
- ½ teaspoon sea salt
- 2 tablespoons fresh lemon juice

Directions

Chop the carrots and parsnips into 2-inch sections and then cut each section into thin sticks.

Toss together the carrots and parsnip sticks with extra virgin olive oil, lemon juice, and salt in a bowl and spread into a baking sheet lined with parchment paper.

Bake the sticks at 425° for about 20 minutes or until browned.

Nutritional Information per Serving:

Calories: 183; Total Fat: 7.3 g; Net Carbs: 22 g; Dietary Fiber: 8 g; Sugars: 10.5 g; Protein: 2.3 g; Cholesterol: 0 mg; Sodium: 319 mg

96. Vinegar & Salt Kale Chips

Yield: 1 Serving
Total Time: 22 Minutes
Prep Time: 10 Minutes
Cook Time: 12 Minutes

Ingredients
- 1 head kale, chopped
- 1 teaspoon extra virgin olive oil
- 1 tablespoon apple cider vinegar
- 1/8 teaspoon sea salt

Directions
Place kale in a bowl and drizzle with vinegar and extra virgin olive oil; sprinkle with salt and massage the ingredients with hands.

Spread the kale out onto two paper-lined baking sheets and bake at 375°F for about 12 minutes or until crispy.

Let cool for about 10 minutes before serving.

Nutritional Information per Serving:
Calories: 234; Total Fat: 16.4 g; Net Carbs: 25.6 g; Dietary Fiber: 4.8 g; Protein: 8 g; Cholesterol: 0 mg; Sodium: 533 mg; Sugars: trace

97.   Roasted Chickpea

Yield: 4 Servings
Total Time: 54 Minutes
Prep Time: 10 Minutes
Cook Time: 44 Minutes

Ingredients
- 2 cups chickpeas
- 2 teaspoons extra-virgin olive oil
- 1/4 teaspoon salt

Directions
Preheat oven to 425°F. Spread chickpeas in a medium baking dish and pat them dry with paper towel; bake, stirring halfway through, for about 22 minutes. Transfer to a large bowl and toss with olive oil, sea salt and pepper; return to oven and bake, stirring hallway through, for another 22 minutes or until dry and golden.

Nutritional Information per Serving:
Calories: 512; Total Fat: 11.2 g; Net Carbs: 17.2 g; Dietary Fiber: 23.2 g; Sugars: 14.2 g; Protein: 25.8 g; Cholesterol: 0 mg; Sodium: 230 mg

98.   Healthy Guacamole

Yield: 2 Servings
Total Time: 10 Minutes
Prep Time: 10 Minutes
Cook Time: N/A

Ingredients

- o 2 cups thawed frozen green peas
- o ¼ cup fresh lime juice
- o 1 teaspoon crushed garlic
- o ½ teaspoon cumin
- o ½ cup chopped cilantro
- o 4 green onions, chopped
- o 1 tomato, chopped
- o Sea salt

Directions

Ina food processor, blend together peas, lime juice, garlic, and cumin until very smooth; transfer to a large bowl and stir in cilantro, green onion, tomato and sea salt. Refrigerate, covered, for about 30 minutes for flavors to blend. Enjoy!

Nutrition Information per Serving

Calories: 137; Total Fat: 0.8 g; Net Carbs: 16.4 g; Dietary Fiber: 8.8 g; Sugars: 9.9 g; Protein: 8.9g Cholesterol: 0 mg; Sodium: 90 mg

99.　Turmeric Nut & Coconut Balls

Yield: 12 Servings
Total Time: 10 Minutes
Prep Time: 10 Minutes
Cook Time: N/A

Ingredients

- 1 cup raw cashews
- 1 1/2 cup shredded coconut
- 1 tablespoon raw honey
- 3 teaspoons ground turmeric
- 1 teaspoon cinnamon
- 1 teaspoon ground ginger
- 1/2 teaspoon sea salt

Directions

In a food processor, process coconut until almost oily; add in the rest of the ingredients and process until cashews are finely chopped.

Press the mixture into bite-sized balls and arrange them on a baking tray. Refrigerate until firm before serving.

Nutritional Information per Serving:

Calories: 110; Total Fat: 8.7 g; Net Carbs: 5.9 g; Dietary Fiber: 1.5 g; Sugars: 2.7 g; Protein: 2.2 g; Cholesterol: 0 mg; Sodium: 82 mg

100.   Apricot-Sesame Balls

Yield: 8 Servings
Total Time: 10 Minutes
Prep Time: 10 Minutes
Cook Time: N/A

Ingredients

- 2 tablespoons sesame seeds
- 1 cup apricots
- 1 cup natural gluten-free muesli
- 1 cup almonds
- 2 tablespoons raw honey
- 1 teaspoon ground cinnamon

Directions

In a food processor, process almonds until finely chopped; add in raw honey, muesli, apricots, and cinnamon and process until very smooth.

Add sesame seeds in a shallow dish. Roll two tablespoons of the almond mixture into bite-sized balls and then roll them into the sesame seeds until well coated.

Arrange them on a tray and refrigerate until set. Serve and store the rest in an airtight container.

Nutritional Information per Serving:

Calories: 163; Total Fat: 8.7 g; Net Carbs: 16 g; Dietary Fiber: 3.3 g; Sugars: 9.1 g; Protein: 4.7 g; Cholesterol: 0 mg; Sodium: 1 mg

101.   Dried Fruit & Nut Mix

Yield: 4 Servings
Total Time: 5 Minutes
Prep Time: 5 Minutes
Cook Time: N/A

Ingredients

- ¼ cup unsalted roasted peanuts
- ¼ cup whole shelled almonds
- ¼ cup chopped pitted dates
- ¼ cup dried cranberries
- 2 ounces dried apricots

Directions

In a medium bowl, mix together all the ingredients until well combined. Enjoy!

Nutrition information per Serving:

Calories: 128; Total Fat: 7.6 g; Net Carbs: 10.4 g; Dietary Fiber: 2.9 g; Sugars: 9.2 g; Protein: 4.1 g; Cholesterol: 0 mg; Sodium: 2 mg

102.   Tahini Dip

Yield: 4 Servings
Total Time: 5 Minutes
Prep Time: 5 Minutes
Cook Time: N/A

Ingredients

- ½ cup tahini
- 1 teaspoon grated garlic
- 2 teaspoons ground turmeric
- 1 tablespoon grated fresh ginger
- ¼ cup fresh lemon juice
- ¼ cup water
- ½ teaspoon salt
- 4 carrots to serve

Directions

In a bowl, whisk together tahini, turmeric, ginger, water, vinegar, garlic, and salt until well blended.

Serve with carrots.

Nutrition information per Serving:

Calories: 222; Total Fat: 16.4 g; Net Carbs: 11.5 g; Dietary Fiber: 5.5 g; Sugars: 4 g; Protein: 6.2 g; Cholesterol: 0 mg; Sodium: 369 mg;

103.   Roasted Pumpkin Seeds

Yield: 4 Servings
Total Time: 25 Minutes
Prep Time: 5 Minutes
Cook Time: 20 Minutes

Ingredients

- 1 cup shelled pumpkin seeds
- 2 tablespoons fresh lime juice
- ¼ teaspoon sea salt

Directions

Preheat oven to 350°F.

Toss pumpkin seeds with fresh lime juiceand sea salt until well coated; spread over a baking sheet and bake for about 20 minutes, stirring once. Remove from oven and let cool before serving.

Nutritional Information per Serving:

Calories: 189; Total Fat: 15.9 g; Net Carbs: 5.1 g; Dietary Fiber: 1.6 g; Sugars: 0.5 g; Protein: 8.6 g; Cholesterol: 0 mg; Sodium: 13 mg

104.   Whole Grain Crackers

Yield: 6 Servings
Total Time: 20 Minutes
Prep Time: 5 Minutes
Cook Time: 15 Minutes

Ingredients:

- 1 cup coconut milk
- 2 teaspoons sesame seeds
- 1 cup whole wheat flour
- 2 teaspoons mixed herbs such as basil and oregano
- ¼ teaspoon sea salt

Directions

In a large bowl, whisk together all the ingredients until stiff dough is formed.
Roll it out into thin chapatis and cut into small strips. Bake them in a 450°F oven for about 15 minutes or until crispy.

Nutrition Information per Serving

Calories: 174; Total Fat: 10.2 g; Carbs: 18.4 g; Dietary Fiber: 1.6 g; Sugars: 1.4 g; Protein: 3.3 g Cholesterol: 0 mg; Sodium: 85 mg

105.   Raw Banana Mash Snack

Yield: 3 Servings
Total Time: Minutes
Prep Time: 10 Minutes
Cook Time: N/A

Ingredients

- 3 ripe bananas
- 1 cup blueberries
- 1 cup diced apple
- 4 tablespoons almond butter

Directions

Mash bananas in a large bowl; serve topped with the remaining ingredients.
Mash the bananas in a bowl, then top with the remaining ingredients.

Nutrition Information per Serving

Calories: 267; Total Fat: 12.6 g; Carbs: 39.2 g; Dietary Fiber: 7.2 g; Sugars: 23.1 g; Protein: 6 g Cholesterol: 0 mg; Sodium: 3 mg

106.   Berry Power Bars

Yield: 10 Bars
Total Time: 45 Minutes
Prep Time: 10 Minutes
Cook Time: 35 Minutes

Ingredients:

- o 1 ½ cups shredded coconut
- o ½ cup dried cranberries
- o ½ cup golden flax meal
- o ½ cup coconut butter
- o 1 cup hemp seeds
- o 1 teaspoon raw honey
- o A good pinch of Celtic sea salt

Directions:

Combine the cranberries, flax, and hemp seeds in your food processor and pulse until well ground.

Add the shredded coconut, coconut butter, honey, and salt and pulse until it forms thick dough.

Transfer the dough to a baking dish and bake for 10 minutes, then remove from oven. Let cool completely, then chill in the fridge to firm up. Slice it into bars and enjoy!

Nutritional Information per Serving:

Calories: 151; Total Fat: 13.6 g; Carbs: 43.2 g; Dietary Fiber: 5.9 g; Sugars: 1.7 g; Protein: 3.8 g; Cholesterol: 0 mg; Sodium: 5 mg

107. Roasted Pumpkin Seeds

Yield: 4 Servings
Total Time: 25 Minutes
Prep Time: 5 Minutes
Cook Time: 20 Minutes

Ingredients

- 1 cup shelled pumpkin seeds
- 2 tablespoons fresh lime juice
- 1 teaspoon chili powder
- ¼ teaspoon sea salt

Directions

Preheat oven to 350°F.

Toss pumpkin seeds with fresh lime juice, chili powder and sea salt until well coated; spread over a baking sheet and bake for about 20 minutes, stirring once. Remove from oven and let cool before serving.

Nutritional Information per Serving:

Calories: 189; Total Fat: 15.9 g; Net Carbs: 5.1 g; Dietary Fiber: 1.6 g; Sugars: 0.5 g; Protein: 8.6 g; Cholesterol: 0 mg; Sodium: 13 mg

108.   Healthy Raw Bars

Yield: 6 Servings
Total Time: 10 Minutes
Prep Time: 15 Minutes
Cook Time: 5 Minutes

Ingredients

- 1/2 cup toasted pistachios
- ½ cup goji berries
- 1/2 cup roasted almonds
- 1/4 cup chia seeds
- 3/4 cup blackcurrants
- 3/4 cup coconut flakes, toasted
- 1 tablespoon turmeric powder
- 1/3 cup ginger
- 1 tablespoon raw cacao nibs
- 1 tablespoon coconut oil
- 500g chopped dark chocolate
- Pinch of sea salt

Directions

Prepare a baking pan by greasing and lining with baking paper.

In a blender, blend together 1/3 cup of pistachios, blackcurrants, ½ cup of coconut flakes, ¼ cup of goji berries, almonds, chia seeds, turmeric powder, and ginger until smooth. In another bowl, stir together cacao nibs, the remaining pistachios and coconut flakes, and the remaining goji berries.

In a saucepan, stir together oil, chocolate and salt until chocolate is melted. Pour the chocolate mixture into the pistachio mixture and stir until well coated; transfer to the pan and sprinkle with the cacao mixture. Refrigerate for at least 4 hours or until firm.

Cut into 24 squares and serve, storing the rest in the refrigerator for up two weeks.

Nutritional Information per Serving:

Calories: 218; Total Fat: 15 g; Carbs: 18 g; Dietary Fiber: 2 g; Sugars: 13 g; Protein: 3 g; Cholesterol: 0 mg; Sodium: 110 mg

109.   Toasted Almonds & Seed Mix

Yield: 4 Servings
Total Time: 20 Minutes
Prep Time: 10 Minutes
Cook Time: 10 Minutes

Ingredients

- 2 tablespoons extra-virgin olive oil
- 1/2 cup sunflower seeds
- 1/2 cup pumpkin seeds
- 1 cup almonds
- 1 tablespoon crushed fennel seeds
- 1 tablespoon ground cumin
- ½ teaspoon sea salt

Directions

Heat oil in a skillet set over medium heat; stir in chili paste and fennel seeds and then add in seeds and almonds; sauté for about 5 minutes and then stir in cumin and salt. Remove from heat and let cool before serving.

Nutritional Information per Serving:

Calories: 347; Total Fat: 30.9 g; Carbs: 18 g; Dietary Fiber: 4.9 g; Sugars: 2.2 g; Protein: 11.2 g; Cholesterol: 1 mg; Sodium: 287 mg

110.   Savory Trail Mix

Yield: 1 Servings
Total Time: 5 Minutes
Prep Time: 5 Minutes

Ingredient

- ¼ cup chopped almonds
- 1/4 cup pumpkin seeds
- 1/4 cup sunflower seeds
- 1/2 teaspoon garlic powder
- 1/2 teaspoon onion powder

Directions

Mix everything and enjoy!

Nutritional Information per Serving:

Calories: 386; Total Fat: 33 g; Carbs: 14.4 g; Dietary Fiber: 9.2 g; Sugars: 3.9 g; Protein: 17.8 g; Cholesterol: 0 mg; Sodium: 331 mg

111.   Almond Coconut Protein Bars

Yield: 3 Servings
Total Time: 10 Minutes
Prep Time: 10 Minutes

Ingredient

- 1/4 cup raw almonds
- 1/4 cup raw hemp seeds
- 1/4 cup medjool dates
- 1 scoop protein powder
- 1/3 cup shredded coconut

- 1 teaspoon melted coconut oil
- 1 tsp. cinnamon
- 1/4 tsp. sea salt
- 1/4 cup water

Directions

In a food processor, process almonds until finely chopped; add in hemp seeds and dates and process to form dough. Transfer the mixture to a bowl and then mix in the remaining ingredients until well blended.

Transfer the dough to a baking pan and press until dough hold together well.

Refrigerate for at least an hour and then cut into six bars. Enjoy!

Nutritional Information per Serving:

Calories: 199; Total Fat: 12.3 g; Carbs: 10.1 g; Dietary Fiber: 7.3 g; Sugars: 2.6 g; Protein: 10.1 g; Cholesterol: 0 mg; Sodium: 101 mg

112.   Herbed Humus

Yield: 6 Servings
Total Time: 10 Minutes
Prep Time: 10 Minutes
Cook Time: N/A

Ingredients
- 2 cloves garlic
- 2 tablespoons sesame seeds, toasted
- 2 tablespoons fresh lemon juice
- 1 cup vegetable broth
- 4 cups cooked garbanzo beans
- ½ cup fresh tarragon leaves, blanched
- 1 cup fresh basil leaves, blanched
- ½ cup fresh parsley
- ¼ cup chopped chives
- Baked potatoes, for serving

Directions
In a food processor, process together all ingredients, except chives and baked potatoes, until very smooth; stir in chives and serve with baked potatoes.

Nutrition Information per Serving
Calories: 523; Total Fat: 10 g; Carbs: 83.5 g; Dietary Fiber: 13.9 g; Sugars: 14.5 g; Protein: 27.9 g Cholesterol: 0 mg; Sodium: 161 mg

113.   Raw Chia-Choco Bars

Yield: 6 Servings
Total Time: 50 Minutes
Prep Time: 20 Minutes
Cook Time: 30 Minutes

Ingredients

- 1/3 cup chia seeds
- 1 ½ cups dates, pitted
- 1 cup, chopped walnut
- 1/3 cup coconut flakes, unsweetened
- 1/3 cup cacao powder
- ¼ cup cacao chips
- 1 teaspoon pure vanilla extract
- 1/3 cup oats
- Sea salt to taste

Directions

Puree the dates in a blender or food processor until pureed. Add the chia seeds, coconut flakes, vanilla, cacao and salt and process until perfectly combined. Transfer the mixture to a bowl and mix in the chocolate, oats and walnuts.

Line a baking pan with wax paper and press the mixture into the pan. Cover and chill overnight.

Cut into bars and store in an airtight container.

Nutritional Information per Serving:

Calories: 161; Total Fat: 2.2 g; Carbs: 37.3g; Dietary Fiber: 4.5g; Sugars: 28.7 g; Protein: 1.9; Cholesterol: 0 mg; Sodium: 41 mg

114. Avocado with Sriracha Snack

Yield: 2 Servings
Total Time: 5 Minutes
Prep Time: 5 Minutes
Cook Time: N/A

Ingredients

- 1 avocado, peeled and cut in two
- 1 tablespoon sriracha
- 2 tablespoons freshly squeezed lime juice
- Sea salt to taste

Directions

Top the halved avocadoes with lime juice, sriracha, and sea salt.
Enjoy!

Nutritional Information per Serving:

Calories: 213; Total Fat: 19.6 g; Carbs: 10.1g; Dietary Fiber: 6.7g; Sugars: 0.5 g; Protein: 1.9g; Cholesterol: 0 mg; Sodium: 59 mg

115.   Carrot French Fries

Yield: 2 Servings
Total Time: 35 Minutes
Prep Time: 15 Minutes
Cook Time: 20 Minutes

Ingredients

- 6 large carrots
- 2 tablespoons extra virgin olive oil
- ½ teaspoon sea salt

Directions

Chop the carrots into 2-inch sections and then cut each section into thin sticks.

Toss together the carrots sticks with extra virgin olive oil and salt in a bowl and spread into a baking sheet lined with parchment paper.

Bake the carrot sticks at 425° for about 20 minutes or until browned.

Nutritional Information per Serving:

Calories: 209; Total Fat: 14 g; Carbs: 21.2 g; Dietary Fiber: 5.3 g; Protein: 1.8 g; Cholesterol: 0 mg; Sodium: 617 mg; Sugars: 10.6 g

116.   Spiced Apple Crisps

Yield: 4 Servings
Total Time: 35 Minutes
Prep Time: 1 Minutes
Cook Time: 25 Minutes

Ingredients
- 4 apples, slices
- 1 tablespoon raw honey
- ½ teaspoon sea salt
- 2 teaspoon cinnamon
- 1 cup virgin olive oil

Directions
In a large bowl, stir together cinnamon, honey, and sea salt until well blended; add the apple slices into the mixture and toss to coat well.

Heat olive oil in a skillet over medium heat; add in the apple slices and deep fry until golden browned. Drain the apple crisps onto paper towel lined plates and serve with a cup of tea.

Nutritional Information per Serving:
Calories: 413 Total Fat: 21.3 g; Net Carbs: 26 g; Dietary Fiber: 6.8 g; Sugars: 22.3 g; Protein: 3.9 g; Cholesterol: 0 mg; Sodium: 321 mg

117.   Healthy Chili-lime Fruit & Veggie Sticks

Yield: 2 Servings
Total Time: 5 Minutes
Prep Time: 5 Minutes
Cook Time: N/A

Ingredients

- 6 spears cucumber
- 6 spears very ripe pineapple
- 6 spears jicama

- 1 teaspoon chili lime seasoning
- 2 lime wedges

Directions

In a bowl, mix together cucumber, pineapple, jicama, lime juice, chili lime seasoning until well combined. Serve garnished with lime wedges. Enjoy!

Nutritional Information per Serving:

Calories: 17; Total Fat: 0 g; Carbs: 4.3 g; Dietary Fiber: 1 g; Sugars: 2 g; Protein: 0 g; Cholesterol: 0 mg; Sodium: 11 mg

118.   Mixed Seed Crackers

Yield: 5 Servings
Total Time: 1 Hour 10 Minutes
Prep Time: 10 Minutes
Cook Time: 1 Hour

Ingredients

- 1/4 cup amaranth
- 1/4 cup flaxseeds
- 1 tablespoon sesame seeds
- 2 tablespoons black chia seeds
- 1/2 cup sunflower seeds
- 1/4 cup pepitas
- 3/4 cup warm water
- 1 teaspoon sea salt

Directions

In a bowl, mix together amaranth, seeds, and pepitas; add in warm water and let sit until all water in absorbed. Stir in salt and pepper.

Meanwhile, preheat your oven to 320 degrees and line a baking tray with paper.

Spread the amaranth mixture onto the tray and bake in the oven for about 1 hour or until golden and crispy. Cut into 20 bars and serve.

Nutrition information per Serving:

Calories: 255; Total Fat: 4.4 g; Carbs: 2.6 g; Dietary Fiber: 2 g; Sugars: 0.2 g; Protein: 2.5 g; Cholesterol: 0 mg; Sodium: 107 mg

119.   Ginger Tahini Dip with Veggies

Yield: 8 Servings
Total Time: 5 Minutes
Prep Time: 5 Minutes
Cook Time: N/A

Ingredients

- ½ cup tahini
- 1 teaspoon grated garlic
- 2 teaspoons ground turmeric
- 1 tablespoon grated fresh ginger
- ¼ cup apple cider vinegar
- ¼ cup water
- ½ teaspoon salt

Directions

In a bowl, whisk together tahini, turmeric, ginger, water, vinegar, garlic, and salt until well blended. Serve with assorted veggies.

Nutrition information per Serving:

Calories: 92; Total Fat: 8 g; Carbs: 4 g; Dietary Fiber: 1 g; Sugars: 0 g; Protein: 3 g; Cholesterol: 0 mg; Sodium: 151 mg;

120.   Cinnamon Mango Trail Mix

Yield: 1 Serving
Total Time: 5 Minutes
Prep Time: 5 Minutes
Cook Time: N/A

Ingredient

- 2 tablespoons chopped toasted cashews
- 2 tablespoons chopped toasted Brazil nuts
- 2 tablespoons toasted peanuts

- ¼ cup dried mango
- 2 tablespoons toasted coconut flakes
- 1 teaspoon cinnamon
- 1 teaspoon cumin

Directions

Mix everything and enjoy!

Nutritional Information per Serving:

Calories: 457; Total Fat: 32 g; Carbs: 34 g; Dietary Fiber: 19 g; Sugars: 13 g; Protein: 14 g; Cholesterol: 0 mg; Sodium: 221 mg

Conclusion

Congratulations for reading through this no gallbladder diet guide and I am confident you have learnt a lot of useful information that is going to have a huge healthy impact in your life.

As you have seen, you can live a higher quality of life with your gallbladder removed compared to when you were fighting gallstones or any other gallstone related disorders. The important thing is before any making any decision, especially within a month of your surgery, consult with your doctor.

Once you are completely healed, embrace a healthy lifestyle of eating natural and healthy foods that have not undergone processing, meditate and exercise at least for 5 days in a week for a minimum of 30 minutes and you are going to live a fulfilling and healthy life.

All the best in your journey and remember to share this book with friends and family and let us help many more people live a perfectly healthy and normal lifestyle with no gallbladder.

Made in United States
North Haven, CT
25 February 2023

33176231R00083